The
Fast
Metabolism
Diet

The Fast Metabolism Diet

EAT MORE FOOD &
LOSE MORE WEIGHT

Haylie Pomroy
Celebrity Nutritionist,
Wellness Consultant

with Eve Adamson

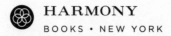

HARMONY
BOOKS · NEW YORK

HAYLIE
POMROY

The material in this book is for informational purposes only and not intended as a substitute for the advice and care of your physician. As with all new weight loss or weight maintenance regimes, the nutrition and fitness program described in this book should be followed only after first consulting with your physician to make sure it is appropriate for your individual circumstances. Keep in mind that nutritional needs vary from person to person, depending on age, sex, health status, and total diet. The author and the publisher expressly disclaim responsibility for any adverse effects that may result from the use or application of the information contained in this book.

Published in the United States by Harmony Books, an imprint of the Crown Publishing Group, a division of Random House, Inc., New York.

www.crownpublishing.com

Harmony Books is a registered trademark and the Circle colophon is a trademark of Random House, Inc.

Library of Congress Cataloging-in-Publication Data
Pomroy, Haylie.
    The fast metabolism diet : eat more food and lose more weight / Haylie Pomroy, B.S., W.C. with Eve Adamson. — First edition.
        pages cm
    Summary: "How to lose 20 pounds in 28 days by jumpstarting your metabolism"—Provided by publisher.
    Includes index.
    1. Reducing diets—Recipes. 2. Weight loss. 3. Metabolism—Regulation. I. Adamson, Eve. II. Title.
    RM222.2.P62 2013
    613.2'5—dc23
    2012042505

ISBN 978-0-307-98627-6
eISBN 978-0-307-98628-3

PRINTED IN THE UNITED STATES OF AMERICA

Book design by Gretchen Achilles
Jacket design by Michael Nagin

20 19 18 17 16 15

First Edition

To my son, Eiland, who taught me that true love was possible, and then came my daughter, Gracen, who taught me that anything is possible. I dedicate this to the two of you.

Contents

Foreword

I t's about time I met you!" Those were the first words I spoke to Haylie Pomroy, the nutritionist at the practice I had recently joined in Burbank, California. Haylie and I had work schedules that didn't coincide, but I kept hearing about this brilliant nutritionist from my patients and the other doctors in the practice. When I finally met Haylie, I had to agree—there was indeed something exceptional about her. Never mind her magnetic personality and the deep caring she obviously has for her patients. The condition of the patients themselves was what stunned me; they were all so happy, satisfied, and on the fast track to health after enjoying significant, even stunning, weight loss through Haylie's program. She was getting results.

I began to refer my own patients to her, especially obese patients with diabetes and hypertension, for whom weight loss was literally a matter of life and death. They would come back to me at their next appointments raving about Haylie and the real, delicious, and satisfying food they were getting to eat. They would even share recipes with me, and so many of them thanked me sincerely for referring them to Haylie. I had never seen such compliance with a diet program before.

At first, after seeing the kinds of results Haylie was getting with her clients, I wondered if this was just another unsustainable weight-loss program that would result in frustration and failure for these patients, many of whom had lost and gained back weight time and time again. But once

Haylie walked me through the program, I began to see that couldn't be further from the truth. Haylie's program is medically sound and grounded in real science, not untested theories or anecdotal evidence. There is nothing mysterious about it. Haylie has an intimate knowledge of how our metabolism works and how biochemical changes triggered by diet can speed it up or slow it down. Best of all, her program works quickly, thoroughly, and the results last. People weren't gaining back the weight.

One of the reasons it works so well is that it is so easy and pleasant to follow. The program uses a system of ingenious meal placement and timing that creates a workout for the metabolism. I've seen weight fall off, cholesterol levels go down, blood sugar stabilize, sleep improve, and depression lift. And not just temporarily—these results have stood the test of time. Haylie always says, "Let food work for you," and she knows how to make that happen, even for the clients whose excess weight has been resistant to other programs.

According to the Centers for Disease Control and Prevention, in 2010, 35.7 percent of adults in the United States were obese, and 34.2 percent were overweight. That means a full 69 percent of U.S. adults weighed more than they should, compromising their health and well-being. Weight problems have reached epidemic proportions, and we have no time to lose. In my practice, I see the tragic side effects: chronic diseases like heart disease and diabetes, depression, and a lifestyle that is less enjoyable and active than it could be. I see patients falling prey to the vicious cycle of radical dieting and binge eating, unable to escape their battles with food and the weight that just won't come off anymore. I also see the psychological cost of weight problems and associated chronic disease, and it is significant indeed.

Haylie provides a light at the end of the proverbial tunnel of diet despair. I wish everyone could meet personally with Haylie because her clients are so fond of her and so motivated and inspired by her. That's why I love that she has finally written a book. Now, anyone can have access to her incredible program and her supportive voice. Haylie uses humor, nurture, and firmness in equal measure to effect changes many of us used to think were impossible. Believe me when I tell you that it *is* possible to make a change in your weight, your health, and your life. I've seen Haylie make it happen, and I can't wait to give a copy of this book to every single one of my patients. The fact that you are reading this now could very well mean you will never have to seek out medical care because of the ravages of diet-induced chronic disease. If I lose a few patients because people are getting healthier, well, that's just fine with me.

So, congratulations! With Haylie Pomroy's help, you and your metabolism are about to start healing.

—BRUCE M. STARK, MD,
board-certified in internal medicine and addiction medicine,
specializing in pain medicine and anti-aging medicine

Part I: Meet Your Metabolism

Introduction

I am the metabolism whisperer.

I know why you can't do it—why your body doesn't respond anymore to the relentless dieting, the mind-numbing exercise, the low-carb or low-fat or high-protein diets. I know why you aren't losing weight . . . and I know how to fix it.

I am a body mechanic, a personal trainer for your metabolism. I'm an innovator, not a duplicator. I've even been accused of adding black magic to my diet plan because the way it works seems so ridiculously easy, and the results defy past experience with other diets. I can assure you that there is no dark magic at work here.

I am out to revolutionize the way people feel about food and use food. You can lose 20 pounds in four weeks by eating real food, never counting calories, and creating a healthy, fast metabolism. There is no magic. There is no con. In meetings, doctors ask my advice and listen. People copy my programs and products, and clients walk out of my office, as my tactful sister sometimes puts it, "Ready to drink the Kool-Aid."

But this Kool-Aid is the kind that really will make you slim and healthy and fabulous . . . and finally free of excess weight. My clients are not people who will be satisfied with a diet that doesn't work, is too hard to follow, saps their energy, or deprives them of pleasure. Those clients include NFL athletes and their wives, as well as TV and movie stars. The Sultan of Dubai even flew in to see me, upon the advice of his physician at Johns Hopkins Dubai.

I've also counseled *a lot* of people who aren't particularly famous but who need to lose weight and lose it *now*, doctor's orders. I have also spent years focusing on face-to-face, one-on-one client care. I consult with intensive weight-loss centers and weight-loss doctors, and I go behind the scenes developing weight-loss programs for major television shows. Advertising agencies and PR firms have flown me out to review their products, from sports drinks for children to healthy lunch programs. I've consulted with Safeway, advised Warner Brothers for their Looney Tunes Back to School campaign, and was on the social-action campaign for the movie *Food, Inc.*

I'm out there promoting health, and making weight loss happen. It's what I do. It's who I am. And it's why I can help you.

I'm telling you all of this so you understand that the Fast Metabolism Diet isn't an untested theory or a product of wishful thinking. I've given this diet to hundreds of clients and seen hundreds of clients lose thousands of pounds, so I know it works. It has to work, or I would be out of business. Instead, all my clinics have waiting lists and people fly me on private jets to their homes just so I can show them how to do this. I'm *your* nutritionist now. With this book, I am taking my program to you. I want everyone who wants to lose weight and get healthier and lighter to be able to do it—fast, effectively, and permanently.

Years of study and clinical work have taught me how to get your metabolism to stand up and pay attention, and how to push it to get busy and start burning away the fat that has plagued you for years. In this book, I'll show you exactly what to do to make it happen for you.

This is not a book for first-time dieters. This is a book for last-time dieters.

It is a book for people whose old tricks don't work anymore. It is for people who love food but who are tired of fighting their cravings, fatigue, and protruding stomachs, and for chronic dieters who just don't think they can diet one more time. If you are about to give up on ever reaching your ideal weight, if you think you must be destined to be heavier than you want to be, then this is your book. Your battle is over. It is time to love food and know how to use it to bring about real, lasting weight loss.

Chronic dieting burns out your metabolism, but the Fast Metabolism Diet stokes the fires again. It works on a simple premise: confuse it to lose it. Just as you might cross-train your physical body to improve your athletic performance, cross-training your metabolism stimulates different burn, build, and restore mechanisms to maximize your efforts.

Through my **systematic rotation of** *targeted* **foods on** *specific* **days, at** *strategic times*, the body transforms itself by cycling between rest and active recovery of the metabolism.

Your body stays surprised, nourished, and revitalized, until it becomes a fat-burning wildfire and the weight finally drops off the way you always dreamed it could. The Fast Metabolism Diet is designed to make you healthier, lighter.

You will eat in three different ways each week—according to Phase 1, Phase 2, and Phase 3. This phase-rotation continues for four weeks, in order to cover every possible biochemical scenario in your body's monthly cycle (that goes for women and men). You will get more out of your food and your body than you ever thought possible. You'll start burning through food and scavenging body fat like never before. You want quick results that last? This is your diet.

You will come away from this book understanding how the body works and why it responds to your actions the way it does. You will never go on a fast. You will never starve. But you will lose weight.

This is not an empty promise. You can do this. I've seen it happen time and time again, for women, for men, for people in their 20s to those in their 70s. I've created clear, precise meal maps that can be adapted for use with every eating population: gluten-sensitives, vegetarian or vegans, and meat lovers. The plan is easy to follow and hard to resist.

Many of my clients jokingly tell me I'm cocky or overconfident when they share their diet horror stories and I tell them they can heal their metabolisms. Then they begin my program and they say it's like we lit a match inside them. I like to tell clients as they leave my office that I look forward to seeing less of them. And I tell them that if they follow the diet, all they have to worry about is finding a good tailor. Because their metabolism is going to be on fire and their excess fat is the fuel . . . and it's burning off, baby.

Get ready to change your life, because food is it.

It's the only thing we have to build our bodies, to create a healthy heart, strong bones and muscles, as well as good skin, hair, and nails. It's what we use to fuel the manufacture of hormones that regulate everything in our bodies. It's not just energy. It's life. It's time to stop being afraid to eat, and learn how to do it the right way. It starts with the burn . . .

FIRE IT UP! IT'S ABOUT THE BURN

Losing weight seems mysterious to some, impossible to others, but it's really not that complicated. It's not about calories or fat grams or carbs. People like to say that losing weight is simply a matter of eating fewer calories than you burn. Calories in, calories out. I've never believed in that, and I've witnessed how untrue it is for some people. It's *not* a matter of eating fewer calories. But it is about the burn.

It's about your metabolism. Fire it up and you'll burn everything you eat like a bonfire, even if you eat a lot. You know those skinny people who always pack it in? They have fast metabolisms. Then there are people who hardly eat at all and remain saddled with extra weight. They are the ones with slow metabolisms that have cooled off and aren't burning the way they should. Tamp down your metabolism until it's like a pile of wet logs, and it's not going to do anything for you. When you throw garbage on a damp pile of wood, it's going to become a heap of wet mess. You can't start a fire with that. All you get is wet logs and moldy garbage. All you get is fat. That's what happens when you throw junk food, processed sugar, and all those other foods you know you probably shouldn't eat, into a body with a slow metabolism. You accumulate fat and more fat and nothing seems to burn.

But you don't want excess fat. You want lean muscle. You want energy, healthy hormones, balanced cholesterol, excellent blood sugar levels, and stunning hair, skin, and nails. You want to radiate health and enjoy the process of getting there. You want to look and feel amazing, but you're sick of depriving yourself.

No problem! Just fix that damp pile of logs. Dry them out, add the right kindling, spray on some lighter fluid, and light a match. Get it burning again, build it into a roaring fire, and you'll be able to eat food like a "normal" person. You'll be able to eat the way you see other people eating, the way you thought you could never eat again.

The problem for many of my clients, and quite possibly you, is that if you are overweight and have spent a lifetime dieting to get it under control (likely unsuccessfully in the long term), the very thing you thought would help you has actually been hurting you. Long-term chronic dieting dampens your metabolism, your inner fire, turning it slowly, year by year, into that pile of wet logs. The less you eat, the more your metabolism cools, and the less you will be able to eat tomorrow.

That's precisely the reason some people can't lose weight even though they don't eat very much. Their metabolic flame has died out, and they can't get it lit again, the logs are wet, the garbage has piled up, and the whole process has become dysfunctional.

They need a jump start. They need to be reignited.

They need what you hold in your hands: The Fast Metabolism Diet.

HOW THE FAST METABOLISM DIET WAS BORN

It all began with a couple of sheep. I'm not kidding! You see, I'm an aggie—that's someone with an education in agricultural science. I was very involved in FFA, Future Farmers of America. I'm a science dork, and my bachelor's degree is not, as you might expect, in food science. It's in animal science. That's where I first began to understand that food can be used, systematically and purposefully, to shape the body the way a sculptor shapes a lump of clay.

I've always been fascinated by how things work, and especially by how the body works. But I was also obsessed with animals, and I thought maybe I could handle the complicated puzzles veterinary science would present. So, at a young age, I decided to be a veterinarian.

In college, my course work was heavily weighted toward animal science. In fact, Temple Grandin (best-selling author, animal science professor, and noted livestock industry consultant) was one of my advisers and a personal mentor. I took classes on sheep production, beef production, livestock feeding, and animal nutrition. I worked as a veterinary surgical tech, and after college, in preparation for veterinary school, I did a nutrition internship at Colorado State. It all added up to an amazing perspective on nutrition. The more I learned about animal nutrition, the more I thought about how some of the same concepts could be applied to people—that diet could be carefully managed to speed up the metabolism and increase the rate of burn in humans, too.

BE A RACEHORSE

I love horses. I ride them and study them and admire them. I also think they can teach us important things about the metabolism.

Some horses are what we call "easy keepers." They do just fine, even get fat, on a small amount of food. Others we call "feed-throughs." You can feed them and feed them and they still have a hard time keeping their weight up.

What's the difference? The horse's metabolism. In animal science, there is a concept called feed-to-gain conversion. How do you feed a steer for the best marbling, distribution of fat, highest grade and pricing of the meat? How do you feed a horse to optimize slow-twitch and fast-twitch muscle fibers, making them faster out of the gate or have stamina for the long haul? Applying these principles to animals, in both the livestock and the horse-racing industries, is a billion-dollar business. So why hasn't anybody been using the hard science we've gleaned from these animals and applied it to human weight gain and loss? It would be revolutionary. So that's exactly what I'm doing for you now.

So which horse do you want to be? The chubby easy keeper or the slim and sleek feed-through? Are you on your way to the Kentucky Derby, or are you going to put yourself out to pasture?

I decided to focus on wellness instead of illness. What if I could help keep people healthy by using my knowledge of animal science? And what if I could do it all by fully integrating my favorite pastime into the mix: food? All this led me to change professional course.

Back in 1995, wellness consulting was gaining in popularity. To become a certified wellness consultant, you must complete a number of science courses, including anatomy and physiology, exercise, nutrition, and stress management, and also be certified in first aid and CPR. This sounded like just the thing for me, so I immersed myself in study. I wanted to be able to assess an individual's health profile and be able to make truly useful, meaningful recommendations about nutrition, exercise, and stress management.

I became a Registered Wellness Consultant specializing in holistic health, nutrition, exercise, and stress management—but then I couldn't stop learning! I went on to garner almost a dozen additional advanced certifications. I loved it. I'd found my calling. I went into private practice as a nutritionist and wellness consultant; and before I knew it, I had several beautiful and bustling wellness clinics: my first clinic, an integrative healthcare clinic in Fort Collins, Colorado; a serene, Zen-inspired clinic in Beverly Hills; a lively Burbank Clinic, located right next to Warner Brothers and Disney Studios and the LA Equestrian Center; and my most recent clinic in Irvine, California, where the focus is specifically on using my nutritionally formulated products to help people lose weight quickly and permanently. (These products *aren't necessary* for doing the Fast Metabolism Diet, but they are convenient if you need them.)

I never advertised my services, but through word of mouth, business boomed, almost from the start. Why? Because of the unique way I use food to shape the body. When you get results, news travels fast.

Many of my clients come referred to me by a network of doctors who know and trust what I do. Many of these clients have chronic health problems like diabetes, celiac disease, thyroid disorders, arthritis, heart disease, or hormonal issues. Many struggle with fertility. All of them need to get healthier so they can heal more efficiently. Healthier patients at healthy weights heal faster. My clients can't just say they feel better; the lab numbers have to change for the better: their cholesterol has to improve, their blood sugars have to improve, their blood pressures have to improve, and so do their numbers on the scale.

And they do change for the better. And the patients keep coming. As my career progressed, business was great, but the more word spread, the more clients wanted to see me personally. My practice has always been very one-on-one. Clients come to see me weekly or every other week, and as they progress, I continue to tailor their programs to their needs. But with the client load I had, this kind of personal service was becoming increasingly difficult.

I began to have clients flying out from hundreds, even thousands, of miles away to see me, or flying me out to their homes to help them. I often went to their doctor's appointments with them and I even cooked with them in their kitchens (in fact, I still do that for some clients). I love that personal contact, but I began to regret that there weren't more Haylies to go around.

I couldn't be everywhere at once, and the people who desperately wanted to work with me couldn't always get to me. I realized I needed to find a way to be there for them even when I couldn't physically be there for them. I needed to craft a system for fast, effective, meaningful, and permanent weight loss that I could send out into the world. So I took the concepts and techniques I used with my individual clients and developed them into this book. I did it so that anyone, anywhere, could follow the diet, and it would work. Quickly. Dramatically.

But there is one catch to this whole "jaw-dropping weight-loss" business: You're going to have to do what I say. You're mine now for the next four weeks, and you have to be willing to accept that. If you really want to lose weight, you have to let me be in charge. You have to commit.

Food can do a lot for you. But it must take a different place in your life for the next few weeks than it probably has up until now. Food is going to wear a different hat. It is your tool, not your entertainment source. It's definitely not your enemy. It is your servant and you are its master. You are going to put it to work for you, and make it work hard. In 28 days, you'll feel a profound difference.

I've been told I can be intense. Bossy, even. However, I'm not being firm with you to amuse myself. I won't be one of those people who encourage you to change your life with vague inspirational guidelines. I will show you *exactly how to do it*. This is a book of action, not theory. Fortunately, it isn't hard. The plan feeds you, both physically and emotionally. It gives you energy, gets you lots of compliments, and most importantly, can change your health.

I can be tough when it comes to the plan, but it is tough love. I care about you. I care about your life and I care about your health. I'm here to help you. Committing to Fast Metabolism doesn't require counting calories, fat grams, or anything else. You want to lose weight, not do math, right? All you have to do is eat food—good food, delicious, real food—in the specific order and way that I tell you to eat it. Give me four weeks and I'll set your metabolism on fire.

I'VE BEEN THERE AND I KNOW WHAT IT'S LIKE

Just in case you are still wondering whether you should go out on the proverbial limb and throw all your trust into my system, let me assure you: I get it. I know what it's like to be overweight and tired, frustrated and cynical, ready to give up. I've been there, personally. I also know what it's like to battle emotions and try to soothe them with food. I know what it's like to go through a divorce, to be a single mom. I know what it's like to try to lose weight under extreme stress; to be sick, to be confused, to feel lost.

But I also know what it's like to get better, lose weight, heal, feel hope, and find my way. I've traveled down that road. And I've done my homework. I'm obsessed with information, and when my clients want to know *why*, I want to know why, too. I've spent years reading endocrinology books, attending advanced medical seminars, learning about hormones and immunology, food allergies, and herbal medicine. If a client wants to know what water to drink, I attend a seminar on water so I can give him, or her, the right answer. I've cultivated a whole network of specialists to support my practice, people from Brigham and Women's Hospital, the Cleveland Clinic, the Holtdorf Clinic, Children's Hospital, the Mayo Clinic, even clinics in Germany and Mexico. I'm not just telling you what I do, though. I'm telling you what science says is *true*, so that it can help you.

A close friend once asked me why I stretch myself so far outside my industry. I joked that I finally found a vocation that allowed me to indulge my neurotic obsession to find out "why." In reality, I do it for *you*. I care about your results. That's the bottom line. I care a lot. I care with passion about all my clients and making sure change happens for them. I want every one of my clients, including you, to be happy and healthy and whole.

So you see, I wrote this book for you. My readers are my clients, too, and what I want more than anything else is to help you effect real, meaningful change in your life. With this book, I want you to become a student of your own metabolism. I want you to understand the health implications of what you're doing as you bring back balance to your body chemistry and increase your internal rate of burn. Foods do different things in the body. Certain foods build muscle; others contribute to fat storage or increase blood sugar. Some provide quick energy. The Fast Metabolism Diet manipulates and enhances your metabolism with specific functional foods combined in different phases to evoke precise physiological changes in your body.

During each phase of the Fast Metabolism Diet, you will notice that you will actually *feel* these changes in your body. By its end, you will understand in a very real and tangible way how your body reacts to foods and how your metabolism can be nurtured instead of bogged down.

This is a diet full of pleasure, not denial. I am going to send you in a new direction, to revitalize your burnt-out metabolism, enjoy food again, rather than fear it or deny it or portion it out on tiny little plates. With the Fast Metabolism Diet, unpleasant diet side effects simply aren't necessary. No starving allowed! You will shake up your metabolism in just the right way to increase your lean muscle-to-fat ratio while enjoying improved health, more energy, and creating a love affair with food.

That is the Fast Metabolism Diet.

So stick with me and enjoy yourself, your food, and your newly emerging body. This is going to be exciting for both of us. Follow the rules and feel the flames of your metabolism rising. You won't be the first. Celebrities trust the diet. Athletes trust it. Rock stars trust it. People with chronic illnesses trust it. Perhaps most important, doctors trust it. You can trust it, too.

So, welcome to my office. Have a seat. I am your nutritionist now and in four short weeks I will be seeing a lot less of you.

CHAPTER ONE

HAYLIE
POMROY

How Did We Get Here?

We are asking more of our bodies than at any other time in the history of civilization. We ask them to live on food that is of a much lower quality than ever, thanks to all the chemical additives, preservatives, and processing. We pump ourselves full of sugar and artificial sweeteners, hormone-riddled dairy products, and foods like wheat and corn and soy that are so genetically modified, it's a wonder we can even digest them. We live in a world with depleted soil, polluted air, and water teeming with environmental chemicals. We eat and drink from plastic containers that leach even more chemicals into our foods and drinks. And, we live with great amounts of often crushing, overwhelming stress.

Given all this, no wonder you don't feel great. You're tired all the time, you get sick too often, or you've gained a few extra pounds (or a few dozen extra pounds). Every day, I see clients who need to make a change in their lives. Some are sick; others are not sick yet, but are headed in that direction. They all need to lose some weight so their bodies can function better. And they need to change now. It's urgent. They feel as if they are wasting precious time—precious days and hours and minutes when they . . . when *you* . . . could feel vibrant and healthy, energetic, strong, and alive.

You want to stop worrying about food and fat and what the scale says to you in the morning. Maybe you've lost a lot of weight in the past—40, 50, 100 pounds or more—but it's creeping back and you're panicking. Maybe you're just so tired of dieting that you're hoping, beyond hope, that there might actually be a better way—a way that would allow you to *eat* again.

I'm sorry that nobody ever *properly* explained to you how your body really works when it comes to food, and how your body chemistry, not you, is to blame. I'm sorry that stress has tipped you into a cycle you feel you can't escape, and you are angry or depressed or even scared about your health and the shape of your body. I'm going to show you another way. The foods you eat and the lifestyle you choose should create energy and strength for you, not fatigue, obesity, sickness, desperation, or self-loathing. Yet once you've slowed down your metabolism, study after study has demonstrated that the metabolic rate does not easily return to normal, even after resuming a normal diet. When you starve yourself, your body adjusts to subsist on a smaller number of calories by slowing down your metabolism. That means that whenever you go off your diet, you're likely to gain weight with a vengeance. Your body is just trying to save you from future famine.

When you are under tremendous stress, your body excretes crisis hormones signaling it to store fat and burn muscle. When you are overloaded with chemicals, pesticides, and pollutants, the body creates new fat cells to house these toxins, so you don't become poisoned and sick. And when you consume food that is devoid of nutrients or contains artificial dyes, flavorings, and sweeteners, the body does its best to survive these foreign substances by slowing down the metabolism and minimizing the damage to the body's system as a whole. The very world we live in puts us all at risk for a slow metabolism.

We're about to change all that. It's time to move beyond blame and regret and self-loathing, and into the future. This is the paradigm shift your body needs, and it will create a new, healthier version of you. The new you views food as a tool to repair damage and restore health. The new you *loves* fruits and grains and protein and healthy fats. The new you knows how the body reacts to specific foods and strategic eating, and the new you has all of the resources to get the weight off and keep it off for good.

We are going to find the new you, and we're going to do it *now*. It's going to take a little work, but it's nothing you can't do. I'm not going to ask you to starve yourself *ever again*. That's likely what got you into this mess in the first place. So let's draw a line in the sand. No more business-as-usual. If food has been your enemy in the past, that's all over. Now, we're stepping into your future, where food is your medicine. Even if you're 10 to 20 pounds overweight, you need this medicine. You need to learn how to **Unwind** stress, **Unlock** fat, and **Unleash** your metabolism.

You wouldn't try to repair a TV or a car without understanding how either is made or functions, and the same should hold true for the amazing biological masterpiece that is you. So first up, let's discuss what metabolism is and does. Then we'll look at some common misconceptions about food and weight loss that may have held you back in the past.

WHAT IS METABOLISM?

This book is all about repairing the metabolism—but what *is* the metabolism, exactly? Metabolism is a *process,* not an object. Specifically, the metabolic process consists of chemical reactions that occur in the cells of all living organisms to sustain life. It's the change or transformation of food into either heat and fuel or substance (muscle, fat, blood, bone). At any given moment, your metabolism is either burning, storing, or building.

You have a metabolism because you are alive, and life requires energy. We all need energy to survive—to breathe, move, think, and react—and the only way to acquire this energy is from the consumption and metabolism, or transformation, of food. Profound! We need fuel, and we need substance. A healthy metabolism and a functional metabolism allow us to have just the perfect amount of energy available, an appropriate amount of reserve energy stored and ready for use, and a strong and stable structure (the body).

YOUR INNER BONFIRE

Before we jump into the nuts and bolts of the Fast Metabolism Diet, let's consider why your metabolism may have slowed down in the first place, and why weight loss hasn't come easy for you.

Remember, your metabolism is your body's system for dealing with the energy you take in through food. The metabolism shuttles that energy into different directions according to what you eat and what you do. The beauty of your metabolism is that it can be manipulated, because how you eat and move and live affects how much of your food is stored as fat, how much is used as energy, and how much is devoted to building the structure that is your body.

This manipulation is what I learned about when I studied animal science. The animal science industry uses this knowledge of energy, storage, and structure to create livestock that is ideally proportioned for use as food, to the tune of billions of dollars of profit.

The metabolism can also get you into trouble because you can inadvertently manipulate it to create a body you *don't want.* Dieting, nutrient-void foods, and living with too much stress slow down your metabolism when it should be sped up. When you gain weight, feel blah, even get sick with a chronic disease, those are all coping mechanisms your body creates in response to your actions or environment, like the frogs that grow three legs in polluted swamps. Your butt or your belly could be protruding because of the very environmental, emotional, and biochemical ecosystem in which it is dwelling.

> **FAST METABOLISM FACT**
> Your metabolism reflects what you do by creating a body that can survive the conditions it is subjected to.

THE SECRETS OF T3 AND RT3

One reason chronic dieting slows down your metabolism is that extreme dieting feels like starvation to your body. Starvation stresses the adrenal glands, which in turn induce a string of chemical reactions in your body that suppress normal production of the thyroid hormones that promote fat burning (T3), in favor of more production of a different thyroid hormone that encourages fat storage (reverse T3, or RT3). This is an oversimplification, but in essence, this fat-storage hormone, RT3, blocks the hormone receptor sites throughout your body, especially in your belly, thighs, and butt, like a goalie defending a goal against the ball. The fat-burning hormone (T3) can't get in there and burn that fat for fuel.

RT3 is a necessary hormone. Without it, we would all have to eat every two hours or we would die. This hormone gets secreted to tell your body not to burn those 500 calories from breakfast or dinner too quickly. It tells your body: "Careful, that might be all you're going to get," or "Don't burn off that whole dinner, you might not get anything else to sustain you until 2:00 P.M. tomorrow!" It's as if someone told you that you had 4 cups of rice and 2 cups of beans to live on for the next month. You'd be darn sure to ration that food so you could survive. You wouldn't want to eat it all the first day. That's what RT3 "sees" when you get too stressed and you don't eat enough: 4 cups of rice and 2 cups of beans.

When your body produces too much RT3, it begins to store fat instead of burn it, even when you have plenty of fat already onboard. As I said above, RT3 acts like a goalie in front of the T3 receptor sites, blocking the ball (T3). Your brain, however, detects the presence of plenty of thyroid hormones, no matter what kind are circulating, so it steps down thyroid hormone production across the board. Your metabolism slows down in response, and then you begin to store *everything* you eat as fat, even healthful foods.

The only way to reverse this process is to jump-start your metabolism again, and the best way to get started is to ditch old, mistaken beliefs about food that are literally weighing you down.

First, let's knock down some of the metabolic myths that are standing in your way, then in the next chapter we'll discuss the five major weight-loss players that we'll fine-tune with the Fast Metabolism Diet before we get to the yummy stuff . . . the food!

METABOLIC MYTH #1: IF I COULD JUST EAT LESS, I'D FINALLY LOSE WEIGHT

One of the biggest misconceptions I hear from my clients is that if they could eat less, then they'd lose weight. In reality, it's exactly the opposite. I can't tell you how many of my overweight clients come to me and tell me that they eat literally no more than 1,200 to 1,400 calories per day.

Often they also exercise five to seven days a week. Yet they still aren't losing weight. They say things like, "I *swear* this is all I eat!" and "I *promise* I'm not cheating!," as if I'm going to send them to the principal's office for food-diary forgery.

I believe them. Why? Because eating less actually makes the situation worse! When your metabolism is too slow, you'll store *lettuce* as fat, and you certainly won't burn any fat. I was explaining to a client the other day that because of the way her body's hormone system was responding, even the carbs found in the beautiful organic mixed greens she was eating were being used as a vehicle to store fat. Shocking and unfair, isn't it? Even the healthiest of foods can do this if your metabolic system needs repair.

This client thought she was doing the right thing by eating so much lettuce, but she'd become so carb-resistant because of years of dieting (as well as the use of diet products, extreme stress, irregular eating, and what I deemed to be an excessive exercise program) that any carbohydrates that found their way into her system, including those in that lettuce, were being converted into sugars and stored as fat instead of being metabolized. Yikes!

I also have clients who skip breakfast, don't eat until 2:00 in the afternoon, then consume 4,500 calories between 2:00 and bedtime. Their bodies have gone into starvation mode by the time they get around to eating. They eat so much because their bodies are panicking and they can't stop themselves. Their bodies are pissed off at them for depriving them of food for so long; they're lucky if it only takes 4,500 calories to calm their bodies again. Why are their bodies reacting so violently by triggering such aggressive eating? When you don't eat until the afternoon, you are asking your body to wake up, get out of bed, shower, get dressed, think, drive, work all day, and sometimes even exercise—all on zero fuel. Talk about cruel.

Guess what else happens when you don't provide your body fuel from food? There's a reason you don't just drop dead when you don't eat. Your body finds food despite you—it finds it in your muscle tissue. It has been proven that a body in starvation mode will first access muscle for fuel, and not fat. So if you do not feed your body, it will "eat" your muscles for the essential fuels it needs to continue life. That's kind of disgusting and more than a little disconcerting to know how key lean muscle is to burning fat,

THE FAST METABOLISM DIET

as well as to keep you structurally fit and able to move with ease and energy through each day.

> **FAST METABOLISM FACT**
>
> Starving yourself does terrible things to your muscles. You know that feeling you get when you're hungry, but don't eat? At some point, you stop being hungry, right? You sure do, but it's not because you didn't eat. You *did* eat. Your body turned to its own tissues for fuel.
>
> This would be great if your body just cannibalized all the excess fat in all the places you don't want it to be. But unfortunately, it doesn't work like that. Instead, the body goes for the muscle first. Because fat is stored for emergencies, your body considers snacking on your own muscle tissue as a preferable option. Yum, bicep sandwich!
>
> Yes, muscle is considered more expendable. Your body's just doing what it thinks is best to keep you alive, yet the result can be devastating for someone trying to lose fat and build muscle. Wouldn't it be better to have a real snack?

Is all that really worth skipping a meal for? And do you really want to fear eating even lettuce—or worse, living only on it—for the rest of your life?

METABOLIC MYTH #2: IF I LIKE IT TOO MUCH, IT CAN'T BE GOOD FOR ME . . . OR MY WAISTLINE

Historically, dieting is about refraining, by limiting portions, forbidding specific types of foods, and reducing or changing the times of eating. Most of my obese clients who are victims of extreme dieting never get to enjoy their food. They eat bland foods and repeat a lot of the same boring meals; often these are (in the case of so-called diet foods) devoid of the nutrients that boost the feel-good hormones in your body that keep you satisfied and vitalized. Not only do they end up hungry, but they're also bored and depressed. Dieting can be such an isolating experience.

Life just isn't as much fun without delicious food. Eating that way is restrictive, it is dull, and it certainly isn't effective, because your natural food-sensing system gets all messed up. So another thing the Fast Metabolism Diet is going to do is to encourage you to use all of your senses in a positive way, to help stimulate your metabolism again and be social and create a community around your new way of eating. Pleasure is powerful and stimulates the secretion of endorphins, reduces stress hormones, increases the metabolism—and it helps fat burn!

PLEASURE: NATURE'S METABOLISM BOOSTER

Stress triggers the metabolism to slow down, and the system senses an emergency and goes into fat-storage mode. Stress can also increase cortisol and minimize the thyroid hormone's effect on the metabolism. Pleasure has just the opposite effect. When you take pleasure in the food you eat, you actually work with nature to speed things up. And bonus: you won't need to overeat.

Pleasure stimulates the metabolism by triggering the adrenals to produce endorphins. These endorphins—what we know as the feel-good brain messengers—stimulate the brain to produce serotonin, a mood-elevating brain hormone that in turn stimulates the thyroid to produce the fat-burning hormone. Talk about a chain reaction.

Pleasure sets off a terrific cascade of events that lower leptin levels, a hormone that makes you hungry. After sex, your leptin levels are lowest. Taking pleasure in food can have the same effect. When you enjoy what you eat, you get a double benefit: you are satisfied and full.

Something else powerful happens when you step away from self-loathing and guilt and enjoy the food you're eating: you start to take better care of yourself. The pleasure, joy, and excitement about your food translates into pleasure and joy and excitement in the choices you make about your food and how you live your life in general.

A client recently sent me this actual text: "I had so much pleasure and excitement tonight! May it all trigger my thyroid to burn that tiramisù I enjoyed so much! LOL, I'll send you my weight in the morning."

To me, the idea of subsisting on poached chicken breasts and steamed vegetables, and *getting fatter anyway,* sounds like torture. If I'm going to go down in a gut-busting blaze of glory, it's going to be with a cheesecake in one hand and ice cream in the other! And you can have cheesecake and ice cream—*if* you stoke your metabolism, getting it burning fast and hot.

When you don't eat enough, your body makes conserving your fat stores a special priority, and it creates more fat from whatever you feed it by secreting special, emergency-only starvation hormones that block fat burning (that pesky RT3). When you eat a lot of nutrient-dense food in the right way, your body relaxes, recognizes the emergency has passed, and starts burning that fat for fuel again—even the cheesecake.

So you have two choices. One, you could just never stop dieting. Eat 1,200 measly calories a day, and cancel your barbecue plans *for the rest of your life!* Because if you ever go off that diet, all hell will break loose. Bam, you're fat again. Just like that. I've seen it over and over. Most of my obese clients have lost large amounts of weight in the past, often many times. Or, two, you can repair your metabolism and live the fast metabolism lifestyle.

PROFILE OF A SERIAL DIETER

Emery is one of my clients, and I consider her to be a typical chronic dieter. A fourth-grade teacher, she was about 30 pounds overweight when she came to see me.

Emery had done all the diets—Weight Watchers, Jenny Craig, the Lindora Diet, and more. She knew exactly how to diet. She knew all the tips and tricks. However, over the years, all the tricks she used to lose weight stopped working. She was eating a low-calorie diet, but had stripped it down so far that it gave her no pleasure and, even worse, it had suppressed her metabolism to the point where she couldn't lose any more weight. She was eating skinless boiled chicken breasts and broccoli. She was eating about 1,200 calories a day. She never snacked. And yet, she was still significantly overweight and the number on the scale wouldn't budge.

I sat her down and told her she needed to go through my four-week program. She would eat five times a day and she would eat the foods at the times and in the order specified.

When Emery looked at the meal map I designed for her, her eyes widened and she looked at me in horror. "If I eat all this, I'll *gain* 20 pounds in four weeks!" she said. "There's no way I can eat all this food."

I told her that if she gained 20 pounds, I would come to her house and cook for her and pack her lunches and load her refrigerator every day. She agreed. Either way, she was a winner. Emery is now down 26 pounds, and she still can't believe it. The last time I saw her, she said, "It's insane. I don't know what just happened to me."

I do. She let her food do the work for her, rather than against her.

In other words, starving (dieting) is bad and e*ating is good*. You remember eating, right? Eating healthy food without guilt? Ring any bells? It's the most important thing I want you to remember. Now say it with me: *Eating is good.*

Eating. Is. Good.

METABOLIC MYTH #3: LOSING WEIGHT IS SIMPLY CALORIES IN, CALORIES OUT

If you're a dieter who has been starving yourself for years, you may still be reeling from the notion that eating is good . . . but I've got another doozy for you.

Calories are a lie.

Here's the response I usually get to that one: "How can you be a nutritionist and not believe in calories?"

Actually, I've probably been in business for as long as I have precisely because *I don't* believe in this old weight-loss equation. When my clients hear that I don't believe in calories, at first they react with disbelief, but soon I begin to win them over. When they realize that calories aren't actually to blame for their problems, that they don't have to count them anymore (since they aren't real), it's like they've been let out of jail. What

THE FAST METABOLISM DIET

chronic dieter wouldn't love to live in a world where calories didn't exist? You *do* live in that world. You might think I'm crazy, and you might even get mad at me for saying it (you wouldn't be the first one), but it's absolutely true. I'll believe that Santa and the Easter Bunny regularly go jogging together in the off season before I'll believe that a chicken breast or a brownie or a tuna salad sandwich has, say, 200 calories. That's like saying that a bodybuilder and my 92-year-old grandma are going to expend the same amount of energy lifting a 40-pound dumbbell.

Of course they won't. That's absurd. And so is the idea that 1 cup of oil-popped popcorn has 55 calories or two slices of pepperoni pizza have 420 calories.

I believe that one of the greatest, most pervasive misconceptions today is the false notion that losing weight is simply a matter of calories in, calories out. It sounds logical, but it's just not true. The calories in/calories out theory is a vast and grossly deceiving oversimplification of how the body uses energy. It is also, in my opinion, a malicious marketing tool that has been used to advocate unhealthy and damaging foods.

A calorie, as used by the food and diet industry, is actually a kilocalorie (kcal), or 1,000 calories, as used in chemistry. (We'll call it a calorie because that's the convention.) A calorie is just the amount of energy required to raise the temperature of 1 kilogram of water 1 degree Celsius, when the food is sealed and burned to ash inside a container surrounded by water.

In school and in clinical practice, I could never wrap my head around the idea of counting calories like they were some little round balls or molecules that made up food. They're not. A calorie is not an object. What does food sealed in a container surrounded by water and burned to ash have to do with you and your body? Nothing.

A calorie is just energy. In food that hasn't been burned (or eaten) yet, it's potential energy. Outside the lab, this potential energy, or "calorie," has very little to do with a food-burning experiment. In the real world, "calories" are subject to millions of variables—since each person has a unique body and biochemical make-up—so a calorie isn't going to be the same thing for you as it is for anyone else. What really matters, much more than the number of theoretical "calories" you do or don't consume, is how you burn the food or otherwise distribute the energy, once it gets inside you.

In the real world, in a real human body, a so-called calorie is just energy potential, and an individual could potentially get fat on 1,400 calories a day, just as she could get fat on 2,400 calories a day. She could also potentially get skinny on 1,400 calories or 2,400 calories a day. It all depends on what the body is doing with the potential energy taken in. If it burns those calories for fuel, then poof! Those calories are used and gone. If it stores them as fat, they sit there, on the hips or butt or belly, still waiting to be used. The idea that 200 calories for you is the same thing as 200 calories for me is ridiculous. So why bother to even think about it that way? It's misleading and depressing, and it pisses me off.

The human body is a complex melding of millions of interrelated chemical processes, and every one of them can potentially affect what happens to the food you eat and the energy you expend, and how it relates to the muscle fibers you gain or lose and the fat cells you accumulate or deflate.

Think of it this way. Say you need to move a car. A car is really heavy, so it's hard to move it. But if I give you a car key, or I show you where you can get a crane, moving a car is easy. If you don't have a key, or a crane, and the emergency brake is on, then, well, you're probably screwed. That car's not going anywhere.

Burning "calories" is similar. Say you need to burn those theoretical 100 calories. If your metabolism is in a state of dysfunction, that's like not having the car key or the crane. Those 100 calories are going to be extremely hard to burn, like pushing that car uphill with the emergency brake on. Good luck with that.

But if you've got the key, which is a fast metabolism fueled by nutrient-rich food, then burning 100 calories is practically effortless. You just turn the key and drive away. That's not to say that someone with a high metabolism can regularly eat 8,000 calories a day (unless he is an Olympic swimmer), but it is saying that when you do have a high-calorie day, your body will be ready. It's important to stoke your metabolic fire constantly, just in case a hot fudge sundae crosses your path.

YOUR BURN RATE

What's really indicative of what will happen to your body when you eat food isn't calories at all, but your *burn rate*, or your metabolism. As I said earlier, your metabolism determines what to do with the food you eat—whether to burn it, use it for building the structure of your body, store it in your liver as glycogen for quick fuel, or store it in pockets all over your body as fat (you know the ones I mean—what collects on your butt, your thighs, and/or your belly).

So many different things influence your burn rate, and they have nothing to do with the number of calories in the food you choose. Do you have a broken leg and your body needs energy for repair? Did you sleep well last night? Have you gone four days without a good bowel movement? Are you dehydrated? Have you moved from that desk chair in the last seven hours? All of these conditions influence how you use calories. Also relevant is the nutrient density and the type of food, and when you eat it and how you eat it, as well as your stress level, activity level, and current body composition or your muscle-to-fat ratio. There's no way to pin it down to a number.

> **FAST METABOLISM FACT**
> Empty calories create empty promises. They do nothing for your metabolism. But nutrient-dense calories rev it up again. Don't worry about calories—instead, consider the content of your food choices.

METABOLIC MYTH #4: DESSERTS MAKE YOU FAT

Don't blame poor delicious chocolate, ice cream, birthday cake, or chocolate chip cookies for your stalled metabolism. Desserts are to be celebrated! When we eat them occasionally with a fast metabolism, we can do so without guilt. When we eat them with a slow metabolism, they stick to us, just like everything else we eat. Add guilt, and you've upped the stress response, elevating the release of fat storage hormones and making the situation even worse. I like to tell my clients that guilt is as fattening as a bag of pork rinds. If you really want dessert, have it with intention and pride and full enjoyment, and most important, *no stress.* If you can't do that, then skip it. It's not worth the price.

METABOLIC TRUTH #1: TO LOSE WEIGHT YOU MUST MAKE PEACE WITH FOOD

Another very important thing I want you to start thinking about, even before you begin the plan, is that if you want to repair your metabolism and reverse the cascade of metabolism-slowing biochemical events caused by stress and chronic dieting, you are going to have to start with one fundamental change: you are going to have to make nice with food again. Your metabolism wants and needs this. It's the way your body is designed to work. So I need you to remember how your body is meant to respond to food.

Each time you ingest food, a series of biochemical reactions takes place. Your body learns what these biochemical reactions are, so that when you smell, touch, or just see a food, your body responds in a specific, learned way and begins responding before you even begin eating. But chronic dieters try to separate themselves from food. They've developed such a negative relationship with food that they've lost all sense of what a healthy relationship with it can be like. I like to say it is the ultimate love affair. This is a relationship that can be hot and steamy, spicy and creamy, icky with sweat and engorged with variety. It also embodies the true meaning of "till death do us part," because without food you will not have life. And without healthy food it is darn near impossible to have a healthy life.

Many chronic dieters see or smell or taste something delicious, and their first thought is: *No!* or *Guilt!* That's not how the body is supposed to react to food.

Let's say you're going to a dinner party; it's a food-centric holiday like Thanksgiving or you're going to your favorite restaurant. What are you going to do? If you're a chronic dieter, you're probably going to feel anxious. *Oh, my gosh, how am I going to handle this? Do I skip the appetizer if everyone else is eating it? I can have one drink but no dessert, or three bites of dessert but no alcohol. I've got to figure out how I can get through the night without eating any carbs.* And worst of all: *I'd better starve myself until tonight, so I can eat everything.*

How can you have any fun at these events if they stress you out? Not only will you be unable to fully enjoy the times in your life that are meant to be enjoyable, but this stress causes fat storage. You'll kick your body into famine mode, and then when you do get to the event or dinner, and you overeat, your body will frantically grab all those calories and turn them straight to fat. You were intending to "be good." To do what dieters are supposed to do. But this is exactly the wrong thing to do unless you want to store more fat, which I'm betting you don't!

We are going to turn that response around. When you've got a fun event coming up, it's much healthier for your metabolism if you were to think like this: *Wow, I got invited to this amazing party! I love Thanksgiving dinner. I can't wait to go to my favorite restaurant!* Then, you need to eat before the event, throughout the day, to get your metabolism going. (I am going to walk you through exactly how to do that later.)

Eating the right way before the big event and feeling positive about it will keep the stress hormones at bay. Instead of saying "Red alert, store every molecule of fat!" your body will say, "Oh boy! Let's get geared up for this! Let's get moving!" Then your metabolism will be roaring, and you'll be in a great position to burn off whatever excesses you might decide to indulge in during your special event. Not insignificantly, you're also a lot more likely to enjoy yourself, but not necessarily by gorging on food. You'll be more relaxed, happier, and the food you do eat, you'll eat with control and pleasure. It's win-win. (I'll talk more about strategies for handling special events in your everyday life in Chapter Ten, "Fast Metabolism Living.")

It's a whole new way of thinking, and a whole new way of living, and you're going to love it. Repair your metabolism, and better yet do it *by eating great food,* and you won't ever have to worry about calories or guilt or special events or anything food-related ever again. So for the next four weeks, put your head down and charge on through, and let this program get your body back on track.

I had one client I'll call Jack. He was a very tall man who was 100 pounds overweight. He wanted to start the program and do it twice over two months. He was desperate to lose weight because his insurance company would not approve a knee surgery until he was at least 40 pounds down. It was during a time when he was extremely busy at work and under a lot of pressure. I told him, "Jack, just take this opportunity and eat exactly what we lay out for you. The plan is easy. Just put your head down and don't look up and do it. Plow through your work and see what happens when you come out on the other side."

Two months later, Jack looked up and he was 55 pounds lighter, and he was pissed at me. "That was supposed to be grueling. I was supposed to be hungry. Why didn't I do this before? What happened to me?"

With his crazy busy schedule and his desperate need for surgery, he didn't even have time to second-guess the program. He was angry that simply allowing his metabolism to heal and ignite fat burning from within had never been offered to him before. He was angry that for so many years he had had such a negative relationship with food. Before finding his way to my office, Jack had spent years of torturous dieting and fasting, only to find himself plagued with excess weight. He has now reached his goal weight, got his knee repaired, and does mud runs and crazy fitness challenges. He still expresses a twinge of frustration to me that his metabolism had been slow for so many years when a Fast Metabolism was a real-life option out there waiting for him to find it.

I get that a lot and it makes me both sad and happy that I get to do what I do every day.

Fall in love with food again and let it support, nurture, and carry you over the threshold to a new paradigm of eating.

METABOLIC TRUTH #2: FOOD IS SOMETHING THAT WAS ONCE ALIVE AND CAME FROM THE LAND, SKY, OR SEA

Things have to be real to be called food in my book. You know, apples, oranges, avocado, chicken, sweet potatoes, pork, shrimp, almonds, mangos. Chemicals, artificial sweeteners, colors, dyes, fat blockers, preservatives, pesticides, plastics, paint thinners, oven cleaners, weed killers, and spider spray just don't count as food.

Have you ever looked up the uses for some of these chemicals commonly found in our "food"? And what exactly is Yellow #5 or Blue #6? What purpose do aluminum, sodium benzoate, quinolone, carmoisine, and tartarazine 19140 serve in a body? I was reading a package the other day and its second ingredient was Sunset Yellow FCF15985 (E110). I wasn't sure if I was to bake, broil, or deep-fry "yellow," so I decided to skip that ingredient for dinner.

Many of these chemicals are designed to add color to your paint or remove stains from your carpets, to build navy ships and bulletproof vests. They are not food! Therefore, they should not be consumed.

Use them to decorate your house and build bombproof shelters, but do not put them in your mouth. The American Medical Society has coined a term for these industrial chemicals found in or sprayed on foods: *obesogens*. These obesogens disrupt normal hormonal balance and inhibit lipid (fat) metabolism. Obesogens can literally make you fat! Sadly, and ironically, most "diet" packaged foods are loaded with obesogens.

Do not eat them. If you still feel the need to ask why and are not concerned that the accumulation of these toxins might someday kill you, then let me give you another little fact to chew on.

PORTRAIT OF A DIETER WHO DIDN'T EAT FOOD

I met Debi because Extra TV was doing a segment in which they wanted me to make over someone's body. Debi couldn't be more all-American—she worked as a special education aide for the school system, and her husband is a sergeant in the local police department. They have a son with special needs and a lot of stress in their lives. On top of all this, Debi had been trying to lose weight for years. She had spent thousands of dollars on diet programs, but because her metabolism had stalled, she would starve herself and if she lost three pounds, she'd view it as a miracle.

I couldn't help but feel so much compassion for Debi. She was a beautiful, warm-hearted person who just couldn't understand why she couldn't get healthy. She was exhausted, tapped out. Even more worrisome, she had high cholesterol and a family history of heart disease. When I met her, she had no idea what she was supposed to cook or eat or even what foods were good for her. She was existing on fat-free, sugar-free foods and 100 calorie preservative-filled snacks! When I showed her my recipes, she said, "But aren't beans fattening? I haven't had a mango in years. Isn't almond butter 200 calories per tablespoon?!"

Her body had paid a heavy price for her years of dieting on chemical-filled diet products disguised as food. She was on cholesterol medicine (the liver breaks down cholesterol; it was too busy dealing with the chemicals to do this job) and feared she might have a heart attack and leave her children without a mother. What mom doesn't secretly share that fear?

I put Debi on Fast Metabolism, and in fourteen days she ate a lot of food and she lost 14 pounds. She also looked ten years younger, and her doctor took her off her cholesterol medication—in just two weeks!

When you eat real food, it is full of nutrients and fiber. Everything in it can be used for some form of good by the body. Chemicals don't have to be filtered out, preservatives don't block nutrient absorption, and additives don't create some bizarre science experiment inside of your body.

I am a nutritionist. All day long I get questions, phone calls, texts, and e-mails asking me if it's okay to eat this or that. Honestly, I say yes to almost anything that is real food. But as your nutritionist you will never hear me encourage you to eat obesogens.

Let's keep it real and fix your metabolism.

CHAPTER TWO

The Five Major Players— And Why They Are Essential to Metabolic Repair

A lot of my training has been in the holistic health world, and many of my colleagues like to talk about the mind-body-spirit connection. They say that without incorporating mind, body, and spirit, you can't be whole. That's all well and good, I suppose, and I agree with it in theory, but I'm also not exactly sure what it means. How do you do it?

As an aggie (my agricultural training rears its head again), I've formulated my own version of this concept. Instead of mind-body-spirit, I like brain-flesh-hormones. It's not as pretty. It's definitely geekier. But to me, it makes more sense.

First, the brain, or mind, is essential for wellness. How do you think about food? How do you decide to create a healthy relationship with food? What choices do you make, consciously, in your life about your health? How do you manage stress? As we discussed in the last chapter, you have to have your head screwed on straight if you are going to change your life, your relationship to food, and your health paradigm.

Flesh is next. You need a strong structure to thrive—dense bones, strong muscles, clean blood, and supple skin. You have to act to preserve and maximize your physical body if you want to feel healthy and strong, as well as burn, build, or store energy according to your actual physical needs—the needs of the flesh.

Finally, hormones are like spirit—you can't see them, but they have a dramatic effect on everything you do, everything you feel, everything you are. The secretion of hormones is what causes everything in your body to be set into motion. They cause your heart to beat and dictate the storage and release of energy in the body. And the proper balance of hormones plays a huge roll in having a fast metabolism.

Another unique thing about the hormones is the way they react to your environment or outside world. For example, if you meet a handsome man or a beautiful woman, your heart may go pitterpat, or if you come across a scary man or an irate woman, your heart may race and feel as if it is in your throat. Those are all hormone interactions that signal a perceived idea to the brain and cause a physiological, or body, reaction. We want to control some of the hormone interactions that are affecting your weight and health, so that your body is working at its optimal.

In order to have wellness, you need all three—brain, flesh, and hormones—to be working in perfect harmony.

In the last chapter, we talked about changing your mindset, and re-thinking your approach to food and dieting. Now let's look at the other parts—the flesh and the hormones. You know what you think, but you don't necessarily know how your liver works, what your thyroid is doing, or whether your hormones are balanced. But you should.

Your body is like a house—a temple, as they say—and you should know what's going on inside this most precious structure, especially in terms of how it relates to what you can actually do to improve your health and achieve a fast metabolism. Let's begin with the five major players.

THE FIVE MAJOR PLAYERS

1. Your Liver
2. Your Adrenals
3. Your Thyroid
4. Your Pituitary
5. Your Body Substance: white fat, brown fat, and muscle

YOUR BODY'S FIVE MAJOR PLAYERS

It's time to get a little more specific about what's really going on inside of your body when you have a slow metabolism. Don't worry; I'm not going to attempt to give you an anatomy class. There are huge textbooks to cover that subject. However, throughout this book I will say things like, "This is liver food" or "We are doing this to support the adrenals" or "Think of all the T3 sites getting excited as you eat this." And I want you to know what I'm talking about. I'm going to ask you to hang in there while I reveal a little bit of my science-nerd side.

I want you to understand what your body is doing so together we can fix what's not working for you—and for it. Stay with me all the way, be an active participant in this process, and when you're done with this chapter and this book, you're going to understand your body a lot better. You'll also have all the tools you need to create the healthy, sleek, optimally functioning body that nature intended for you.

YOUR LIVER

Your liver is vital and essential to keeping you and all your bodily systems up and running. Over 600 known metabolic functions happen via the liver, and virtually every nutrient, every hormone, every chemical must be bio-transformed, or made active, by the liver. It's your workhorse, and without it, you'd buy the farm.

Your liver creates bile, a nasty-sounding but powerful solution that breaks down fats (and the nitrites and nitrates in your deli meats and bacon). Hormones get secreted from glands all over your body, but it is your liver that breaks down the hormones and makes them biologically active so they can go to work for you. It flips the light switch once you've put in the bulb.

Your liver influences your electrolyte balance, swelling and inflammation, dehydration, bloating, and water weight. It also acts like a filter for the blood that travels through the digestive tract. It converts B vitamins into coenzymes, and metabolizes nutrients such as proteins, fats, and carbohydrates.

Your liver also manufactures carnitine, which takes fat and escorts it to the mitochondria—your body's little power centers or fat converters. The amount of carnitine in your system dictates how much fat can be delivered and incinerated. *This simple relationship between the liver and the mitochondria can influence up to 90 percent of your fat burn, dictating your metabolic rate.* The faster and more efficiently you produce carnitine in your liver, the faster and more efficient your metabolism is.

The food you eat must feed your liver rather than tax it. If you don't feed your liver appropriately and frequently to stimulate it to its most efficient functioning, everything else will get disrupted. Because the liver is so closely linked with metabolism, it is one of the most crucial organs we'll be nurturing with the Fast Metabolism Diet.

YOUR ADRENALS

Your adrenals are small glands that lie on top of your kidneys in your lower back, and they secrete hormones that regulate your body's response to stress of all types: physical, emotional, environmental, and mental. Your adrenals are responsible for the hormones that allow your body to adapt either functionally or dysfunctionally to changing situations. These hormones determine how you access fuel in your body and what you do with the fuel or food you consume. Do you store it as fat? Or do you burn it as energy?

Let's say you have to pull an all-nighter, getting changes on your book back to an editor. Do you continue to feed yourself every three hours, fueling your body, your hormones, and your brain, or do you stop eating at 6 P.M.? That's what you would normally do, even though you aren't sleeping. Answer: When you are awake and working, you have to keep eating. Otherwise, you leave your body without fuel, and then it thinks you are starving and before you know it, your metabolism is slowing down.

Some of the metabolism-specific hormones the adrenals release include cortisol, adrenaline, aldosterone, and epinephrine. These are released in response to stress and/or pleasure. The stressors could be as major as a car accident or as minor as missing a meal. The adrenals respond to the acute stress of a disaster just as they respond to the chronic stress of a bad relationship, an unpleasant work environment, or a taxing family situation.

The secretion of these stress hormones regulates the release of glucose or sugar from the muscle and liver cells, to either stimulate or slow down your body's metabolic rate. That means this process is nutrient-dependent, or dependent on the food you do or don't eat. When you experience stress, the surge of hormones you experience will be influenced by what you've just been eating. If you nourish your body during times of stress with the right foods, you will not store fat as much as you burn it.

To put it more simply, stress pulls nutrients from the body from places where you can't afford to lose them (like muscle). If you are eating a healthy, nutrient-rich diet, your body won't have to resort to this. You'll be able to handle the stress. If, however, you aren't eating enough, or enough of the right food, your metabolism will slow down, due to a complex chain of chemical reactions. If you are eating the right food at the right time, you will feed your adrenals so they can survive the stress without resorting to a slowed metabolism.

Adrenal exhaustion can occur when a body has been under significant stress for a long period of time. This occurs because the body has been chronically secreting stress hormones that are meant to be preserved for quick crisis situations. You know that surging feeling you get when you are startled or scared? That's a hormone surge. I like to think of those fight-and-flight hormones as sacred. They should be saved for a true emergency, but many of us live and survive on the energy from these hormones, day in and day out. That is not the way our bodies are meant to work! When stress hormones constantly surge, the body is constantly in a state of crisis. One of the things that occurs in this situation is that the hormones slow the burning of fuel because the body sees no end to the exhausting demand. Adrenal exhaustion is a problem I'm seeing more and more often in my clinic. Exacerbating this situation is decreasing food quality and increasing environmental chemicals. That's why it's so important to feed yourself clean (i.e., organic whole) food as much as you can. Your adrenals will thank you.

Preserve your adrenals! Soothe them with this diet and stress management.

Let's take a closer look at exactly what happens when your body perceives stress. First, the hypothalamus (an almond-sized gland in your brain) stimulates the pituitary gland (a pea-sized gland at the base of your skull) to secrete a hormone called ACTH. ACTH stimulates your adrenals (those little guys in your lower back, just above your kidneys) to produce cortisol. Still with me? The cortisol, in turn, stimulates the hypothalamus, part of the brain, to tell the pituitary, part of the brain, to slow the production of TSH (thyroid-stimulating hormone).

TSH lowers the output of other fat-burning T3 thyroid hormones, which cause excess formation of fat-storing, metabolism-slowing RT3 hormones. In the absence of proper nutrition, this whole process causes the adrenals to stimulate aldosterone, another hormone, to break down the muscle for fuel (in the form of glucose stored as glycogen), and then to act with RT3 to aggressively convert the glucose into fat, to be stored. This is not looking good for you and your efforts to lose weight and feel good!

If you have an ample supply of amino acids (such as taurine) from protein, as well as minerals like iodine, complex sugars, and a healthy enzymatic liver function (which is dependent on nutrients from food), then instead of cannibalizing muscle for crisis fuel, you can maintain a healthy cortisol secretion response. This will cause T4 to be converted to biologically active, metabolically aggressive, fat-scorching T3 instead of that pesky RT3 that causes so many problems when you make too much of it. Your body will act as a lean, mean fighting machine rather than a fight-or-flight mess of panic and fat storage.

YOUR THYROID

The thyroid is a metabolic superstar! It is a butterfly-shaped gland located at the center of the throat, and although I know I'm mixing my metaphors here, I think of it as your body's furnace. The pituitary gland in the brain (which will be discussed more thoroughly in the next section) is like the thermostat, and the hypothalamus in the brain is like the guy controlling the thermostat. But the thyroid is the furnace and the hormones it produces, like T3 and T4, are the heat. When it gets too hot, its thermostat has to be turned down, and when too cold, its thermostat gets cranked up. If any of these three mechanisms isn't working just right, then the body's temperature—a direct reflection of metabolism, or the rate at which the body is burning energy—will be off. The house will be too hot or too cold.

The thyroid performs many metabolic tasks via many functions in the body, including the extraction of iodine from food to produce the thyroid hormones T3 and T4. The T3 and T4 travel through the bloodstream and influence the metabolism through the conversion of oxygen and calories to energy. This is huge! This is what you want—an efficient furnace fueled by food and heating your house so it's toasty and comfortable. T3, in particular, is the superhero of a fast metabolism. T3 possesses approximately four times the metabolic hormone strength of T4.

But the thyroid has a dark side—a hormone called Reverse T3 (RT3). I introduced you to RT3 in the last chapter, but I want to bring it up again because it's so important in the process of metabolism repair. RT3 is sort of like that dysfunctional family member who shows up at Thanksgiving but doesn't behave and inevitably ruins everybody's dinner. It's a misshaped thyroid hormone that isn't very efficient in stimulating the metabolism, and in fact, it blocks healthy T3 functioning. RT3 doesn't mean to mess things up for you and your plans for those skinny jeans. It's actually a smart response to prevent starvation. The problem is, when you diet, you know you aren't really starving (even though on some diets it might seem that way), but your body doesn't have the 411.

In situations when you are experiencing chronic stress, certain disease processes, or nutritional deprivation, RT3 heeds your body's "Red Alert!" This signals the RT3 to bind to the T3 receptor sites and run interference so T3 can't do its job. RT3 throws a big bucket of water on your metabolic fire, in a panicked effort to save your fat stores so you don't die from what surely must be a catastrophic event or famine. The result is that your body quits burning and starts storing. Sometimes there are serious problems with the body's thermostat, such as Hashimoto's disease, Graves' disease, or a body that is producing thyroid peroxidase (attacking its own thyroid). These thyroid-based diseases are often undiagnosed and can play a very large role in an extremely slow metabolism.

The Fast Metabolism Diet is designed to nurture and coax the right hormone production from your thyroid. But because things can go wrong with the thyroid, I strongly believe it is important to look at the blood chemistry of the thyroid to be sure it's functioning properly. A lot of women's health books talk about the thyroid because hypothyroidism is an often undiagnosed condition that can cause a slow metabolism, weight gain, hair loss, brittle nails, constipation, headaches, and fatigue. I always recommend my clients get thyroid tested (I'll talk about which tests at the end of this chapter).

YOUR PITUITARY

I briefly mentioned the pituitary in the previous section, but let's give it some love. I think of the pituitary gland as the body's thermostat. It secretes hormones that regulate or adjust the actions of many other hormones in your body.

For example, the pituitary stimulates the thyroid to secrete its hormones with thyroid-stimulating hormone, or TSH. If the TSH level is high, that means the thyroid is requiring a lot of motivation or pushing to get its job done (hypothyroid). Imagine the pituitary yelling at the thyroid: *Get going, you slacker! Move it or lose it!*

If the TSH is normal, all the pituitary has to do is speak in a normal voice: *Keep up the good work.* If the TSH is very low, then the thyroid gland may be overactive (hyperthyroid), and the pituitary may only whisper. Of course, as I've explained earlier, if the thyroid is producing a lot of fat-storing RT3, the pituitary may perceive this as plenty of thyroid hormone, and may only whisper when it should be yelling. For this reason, a normal thyroid test isn't necessarily indicative of optimal thyroid function, as it won't separate out the RT3 from the furnace-stoking T3.

The pituitary also regulates sex hormone production, such as estrogen, progesterone, testosterone, and DHEA. The regulation of each of these, as well as the adrenal hormones, is crucial to the health of the body and speed of the metabolism. So the pituitary is not only the furnace's thermostat but also the control center for the huge ecosystem called your hormones.

YOUR BODY SUBSTANCE

The final key player that directly influences the metabolism is your *body substance*—how I refer to the fat, bone, connective tissue, and muscle in your body. The body stores the majority of your reserve fuel in either muscle or fat. Because muscle is constantly contracting, relaxing, beating, pushing, and pulling, it takes a lot of fuel to create and maintain it. This is why they say muscle consumes more calories, or energy, than fat. Fat just sits there. Have you ever seen it do anything besides flop over your waistband or jiggle around on your thighs? Fat really doesn't do much but hold on to fuel, and therefore it takes very little fuel or calories to maintain it. (And remember, if you don't eat or provide outside fuel, the body will actually break down muscle and store some of that fuel as even more fat!)

There are two basic types of fat in the body: white fat and brown fat. For decades scientists believed that brown fat was only present and important in infants and small children, to help keep them warm and maintain their body temperatures. It is now believed that even though it exists in very small amounts in adults, brown fat plays a crucial role in the regulation of blood sugars and the metabolism. Brown fat is brown because it is rich in mitochondria (remember those little parts of the cell that burn fuel and produce energy?).

The more obese you are, the less brown fat you will have and the more white fat you will have in storage (the fat you don't like when it jiggles). This is just another sick joke on your body, because brown fat burns fuel nine times faster than white fat. So why does your body seem so in love with white fat, hoarding it like a miser? It's because your body thought it might need the fuel reserves! (Thanks a lot, chronic dieting!) White fat's major purpose for being is for long-term fuel, and your body will make a Herculean effort to hold on to it, just in case of disaster.

White fat isn't all bad. In fact, you need it and it serves a very important function. White fat is the fat under your skin (subcutaneous fat) and around your organs (visceral fat). It is designed to maintain body temperature, protect the organs, and act as an energy storage site for future need. White fat also secretes some hormones and regulates the output of others, and these hormones communicate directly with the adrenals, the pituitary, and the hypothalamus.

However, when your metabolism slows down, your body goes into super white-fat production mode, hoarding fat like some people hoard newspapers, shoes, junk mail, or stray cats. You can literally be buried alive with all this saved energy in the form of smothering white fat.

Brown fat, on the other hand, is a thermogenic or furnace fat. Unlike white fat, instead of storing energy, brown fat seems to prefer to burn through it. It also helps stimulate the metabolism by warming the body, increasing blood flow, and making it easier to deliver nutrients to the white fat. Brown fat helps regulate your cholesterol and triglycerides, transports waste to the intestines for elimination, synthesizes proteins, and stores and metabolizes fatty acids used for energy. Brown fat also metabolizes and stores carbohydrates, storing them as glucose for your red blood cells and brain.

Interestingly, in adults, brown fat is typically located only behind the shoulder blades up and around the neck and under the collar bone. This is also where I and many of my clients say they feel or hold their stress. Stress hormones directly affect brown fat activity. Brown fat can be your best friend when you want to enhance your metabolism because, through its hormone activity, it releases a ton of energy from food. Brown fat also seems to be activated by cold, while the release of stored energy in white fat seems to be stimulated by heat. Both the burn of energy in brown fat and the release of energy from white fat are supported by healthy thyroid function.

Let's revisit the five major players for a moment, because they are the keys to using food to sculpt your body the way you want it. Feeding your liver, soothing your adrenals, maximizing pituitary and thyroid function, and tweaking your fat balance—all of these are the cornerstones of a Fast Metabolism.

Simply changing the way you eat will mobilize and facilitate healthy hormonal responses to stress, boost the metabolism, and maximize the body's efficient and balanced distribution of fat, water, and muscle. In a very short time, you'll be able to behold the amazing power of food, right in your own mirror!

YOUR DOCTOR'S ROLE IN STOKING YOUR METABOLISM

"How do I know I have a slow metabolism?"

This is one of the most common questions I get, and it's the key reason I like my clients to get some basic tests before they embark on the Fast Metabolism Diet, to see just how out of balance they are. The tests aren't necessary to benefit from the Fast Metabolism Diet, but they can help you to understand exactly where you are and how far you need to go.

I recommend these lab tests with a caveat: they are just one part of that peek into the window of the house that is your body. Imagine you're shopping for a new home. One day, you see a cool house, and you wonder if you should call the Realtor and get a tour of the inside. Before you bother to make the call, maybe you sneak into the yard and take a peek through the window. You see a beautiful living room with vaulted ceilings, hardwood floors, and lots of light. Great! But you can't view the whole house. The upstairs might be completely trashed, with squatters and rats and graffiti on the walls. Or, the upstairs might be fine. You can't tell, because you can't see everything. You can't learn everything about your health from lab tests, but you can get a preliminary picture.

Also, keep in mind that even if all your tests look great, if you are overweight, out of shape, and eat a poor diet, then your body is doing the very strenuous job of maintaining normal body chemistry under adverse circumstances. I've had patients come to see me, and they show me their labs and they say, "Look, everything is normal. I'm fine! The doctor sent me on my way." I can't help saying, "But look! You aren't fine! Just look!"

It's so frustrating when you are overweight and your doctor tells you, "Your numbers are great, you're fine; see you next year." Some of my clients tell me how angry this makes them. "Are you looking at me?" they want to yell. "Do you not *see* me? I am manifesting metabolic dysfunction on my ass!" And they are. So just remember: labs are a peek in the window, but they aren't everything because you don't need a measurable disease to have a slow metabolism. Also, you can have significant symptoms and fall in the "normal" range. You might have perfect labs and a trashed metabolism. If you have more than 10 pounds to lose, your metabolism isn't what it could be.

So why bother to test at all? Because some basic tests can alert you to health problems you might not know about, or might tell you that you're doing pretty well and you really only need a little kick in the pants. Labs aren't the whole picture, but they can provide you and your doctor with some helpful hints.

And speaking of your doctor, this is the time to partner with a doctor who is open to your efforts to lose weight and boost your metabolism, if you don't already have one. There are many great doctors out there. I'm in a unique setting in my offices because I work with some of the most amazing doctors every day, and I have access to a lab right in my clinic. This might not be so easy for you. If your doctor balks at doing tests, tell him or her that your nutritionist requested them. Some labs will now do tests for patients without a physician referral, so that's another option, if it's available to you. None of the tests I mention below are particularly expensive or unusual.

TEAM BUILDING

When I first began practicing in the natural health industry, nutrition fell into the category of "alternative medicine," and I noticed a real us vs. them mentality on both sides of the aisle—from both holistic practitioners and conventional doctors. I never subscribed to this kind of thinking, and fortunately, I see it changing. More conventional doctors are open to holistic methods, and more holistic practitioners partner with conventional doctors in the interests of their patients.

I always felt that everyone and anyone could potentially be a partner in getting my clients on the road to health. One of my mentors, Dr. Jackie Fields, used to say, "It's in the patient's best interest to have a clinic without walls." She meant that if you don't have the answers in house, go out and find someone who does. Create a healthcare team that supports your quest for a healthy and fast metabolism, solid nutrition, and stress relief. You're the team captain. Go team!

The main thing I look for in tests, beyond abnormal numbers, are numbers that indicate a fast metabolism because "normal" test results are typically pretty wide. Knowing your numbers will tell you whether you have the chemistry of a person with a slow metabolism, or the chemistry of a person with a fast metabolism, or whether you fall somewhere in the middle.

Keep in mind that I am not a doctor, so my opinion of what test results indicate a fast metabolism may differ from what your doctor would say. However, I'm not some random person telling you to bug your doctor for pointless tests. These are the numbers I use with my clients at the clinic, and most of them are referred to me by physicians. I request these tests for my patients every day, and doctors often ask for my input on test results because I look beyond "normal" for ideal metabolism numbers, specifically when wanting to facilitate healthy weight loss.

These are the tests I'd like you to ask your doctor to give you:

THYROID: Ask your doctor to test your TSH, T3, T4, and Reverse T3. Don't forget to ask for the Reverse T3 (RT3), as it isn't always part of a typical thyroid panel. These numbers can uncover thyroid issues you might have, but there are a few additional ones such as TPO or Anti Thyroid Antibody they might want to consider if worried about Hashimoto's or Graves'. If these are off, it can tell you even more about your overall health and how crucial it is to nurture your body and its metabolism. If you have a *fast metabolism*, your numbers should look like this, so this is what we will be aiming for:

YOUR BODY'S CHEMISTRY

	NORMAL	FAST METABOLISM
THYROID PANEL		
TSH	.4–.4.5 mIU/L	Under 1.0 mIU/L
T3	2.3–4.2 pg/ml	3.0–4.2 pg/ml
T4	0.7–2.0	1.5–2.0
Reverse T3	90–350 pg/ml	120 or lower pg/ml
LIPID PANEL		
Cholesterol	125–200 mg/dl	165–185 mg/dl
Triglycerides	Less than 150 mg/dl	75–100 mg/dl

	NORMAL	FAST METABOLISM
HDL ("good" cholesterol)	Greater than 46 mg/dl	70 or higher mg/dl
LDL ("bad" cholesterol)	Less than 130 mg/dl	100 or lower mg/dl

SUGAR PANEL

Hemoglobin A1C	Lower than 6.0	Lower than 5.4
Fasting Blood Sugar	65–99 mg/dl	75–85 mg/dl*

ACCESSORY HORMONES

Cortisol	5–23 mcg/dl	8–14 mcg/dl
Leptin	18	10–12

LEPTIN LESSON

Leptin is a hormone that promotes white fat storage, and is typically stimulated by fat-cell production, creating a vicious cycle of fat production. Leptin actually blocks receptor sites for sex hormones, including estrogen, progesterone, and testosterone. When that happens, the body starts storing the hormones instead of using them, and this encourages fat storage. For example, when the body stores estrogen, you might experience bloating and aggressive weight gain. Before we take cows to slaughter, we give them a bullet of estrogen, inducing rapid weight gain and water retention. For we humans, stress, skipping breakfast, and hormone fluctuations that occur during pregnancy, menopause, and even manopause (male menopause) are the most common causes for an increase in leptin. Some of these things are out of our control, so we have to do everything in our power to keep the hormones balanced by the pituitary, metabolically converted by the liver, and readily available to build muscle and not store fat.

We also want to soothe the adrenals by using food as fuel. This is exactly what the Fast Metabolism Diet is designed to do. Control what you can, create an environment conducive to a fast metabolism, and heal the imbalances that have accumulated. You can at least control your breakfast . . . so eat it!

*If it's into the 70s, you are burning fat like crazy!

ESTROGENS: For women only. I think it's a good idea to test your estrogen level at any age. If you are going through perimenopause, that period of up to ten years before menopause, your estrogen levels can reveal if a hormone imbalance can be causing some of your symptoms. Before then, it's a good idea to get a baseline reading so you know when things are getting out of balance later. Ideally, we look at three different forms of estrogen: estradiol, estriol, and estrone. Estradiol is the one most doctors like to monitor. With excessive midsection weight gain or in postmenopausal women, I look at estrone because estrone production isn't just limited to the ovaries. It can be stimulated by fat cells and the adrenal glands, and can be related to stress-related weight gain.

There are many schools of thought on what ideal levels should be for these three estrogens. For metabolism purposes, I want to make sure all three fall into the "normal" ranges, and one or more has not gotten out of control. If you are having a period, make sure to have this test taken as close to day three of your period as possible. This is one of the most accurate times to look at your hormones.

TESTOSTERONE: For men only. Normal could be 200 to 800, but men with fast metabolisms can have numbers as high as 800 to 1200. I like to see 600 or higher. Knowing your numbers empowers you to see one important picture of your current health condition and do something about it—and the thing you can do is to *eat*. The Fast Metabolism Diet is designed to provide the fuel needed for a healthy body. Food is the medicine.

When your numbers are off, when your metabolism is suppressed, change your diet first! You can beat a horse until he reaches the finish line, or you can feed and train and care for him. Either scenario might result in winning a race on that one day, but if you beat the horse long enough, he will break down, slow down, crash, and burn—just when you need the prize money the most.

There are no guarantees in life or health, but the better you care for yourself, and the healthier your metabolism, the more reliable your body's systems will be for detoxifying, eliminating, burning fat, maintaining a healthy body weight, finding healthy hormone balance, and preventing disease.

Nourish and flourish! That's what I want for you. It all begins with a healthy, optimally functioning metabolism. Are you ready to begin exploring exactly how to get one?

Part II: How the Program Works

CHAPTER THREE

HAYLIE
POMROY

Unwind (Phase 1), Unlock (Phase 2), and Unleash (Phase 3): Three Distinct Phases, One Powerful Week

Now you know what can go wrong when you chronically diet or eat foods that don't contain dense nutrition. So what do you do about it? How do you make it right?

When your metabolism has become dysfunctional, it needs the equivalent of a personal trainer to get it back into shape—someone who can take the raw materials of your body and sculpt them into the body of your dreams. Consider me that trainer and Fast Metabolism your guide to cross-training your metabolism.

What do I mean by that? If you do only one kind of exercise, like running or the elliptical trainer, your body gets used to that exercise and you soon stop seeing results. You hit a plateau. You're using the same muscles in the same way every day and neglecting all the other muscles in your body. In the same way that cross-training shakes up that routine by keeping your body surprised, Fast Metabolism shakes up your dietary patterns by doing two things:

1. Flooding you with some of the vital nutrients you've been missing, but never in the same way for more than two or three days in a row

2. Asking your body to do something difficult, but never for more than two or three days in a row

This strategy keeps your body working, surprised, and supported, reversing the biochemical patterns that have slowed down your metabolism. It's your body's wake-up call, and it will trigger a burn that will torch calories and fat like never before.

Cross-training your metabolism also means switching up your meal maps (you'll find out more about those soon!), so the new you will never get in a rut or get bored. Two days eating one way, two days eating another, and then three days eating a whole new, specific nutrient mix. It stimulates the metabolism, it keeps eating interesting, and it works.

It's not a trick. It's just the way nature is. It's a basic principle of physics: a body at rest tends to stay at rest unless something compels it to move. A body in motion tends to stay in motion unless something compels it to stop. This is the same for your metabolism. Once you coax your metabolism into motion, it's easier to keep it moving. You're taking that horse by the reins and walking him around the paddock so you can move him into the trailer.

Now all you need to do is learn how to do the coaxing.

THE FAST METABOLISM DIET—THREE DISTINCT PHASES, ONE POWERFUL WEEK

THE THREE PHASES AT A GLANCE

Phase 1—**Unwind** Stress and Calm the Adrenals
Days 1 and 2

Phase 2—**Unlock** Stored Fat and Build Muscle
Days 3 and 4

Phase 3—**Unleash** the Burn—Hormones, Heart, and Heat
Days 5 to 7

Let's consider how the three phases of the Fast Metabolism Diet coax your body to burn fat, build muscle, balance hormones, and lay the foundation

THE FAST METABOLISM DIET

for a healthier you. Our bodies require variety from our diets in order to get all of the nutrients necessary to perform all biological, physiological, and neurochemical functions. That's just what the three phases of Fast Metabolism give you. You need complex carbohydrates, natural sugars, protein, fat, and even salt to maintain normal body chemistry. At times you need very high therapeutic levels of these elements, especially when you've been depriving yourself for too long. Including these fuels, but not all at the same time, helps you to rebuild, restore, enrich, and replenish your depleted body and your burnt-out metabolism.

Each phase only lasts for a short time so you don't exhaust any one system or part of yourself. Doing any phase for too long is like asking you to clean your whole house when you didn't get any sleep the night before; you'll be exhausted and you won't do as good a job of it. We're going to clean *your* house (your body) room by room, a little at a time, until it's sparkling.

For four weeks, you will follow a three-phase rotation. Each phase is strategically designed to work and rest different body systems, and each has a chance to work during every week of your body's natural 28-day cycle. By segmenting out the work in this way, your body will get all the attention and support *and* high expectations it needs, one phase, or a couple of days, at a time.

When you move through to the next phase, the systems and organs you engaged in the previous phase get to relax, rest, and restore. A healthy metabolism wants to do three things:

1. Take your food and turn it into energy

2. Release stored fat

3. Turn newly released stored fat into energy

Each of the three phases accomplishes these steps when done in order.

Before you can use your food for energy, you first need to calm your adrenals. And that's what the first phase is all about: unwinding.

THE BASICS

This is the high-glycemic, moderate-protein, low-fat phase.

High in carbohydrate-rich foods such as:

Brown rice	Brown rice pasta
Oatmeal	Spelt or brown rice tortillas
Quinoa	Rice milk
Wild rice	

High in natural sugars such as:

Mangos	Pears
Apples	Pineapples
Figs	Strawberries
Peaches	Watermelon

High in B and C vitamins such as:

Lean beef	Oranges
Turkey	Guavas
Oatmeal	Kiwis
Lentils	Lemons and limes

Contain moderate amounts of protein

Low in fat

HOW TO EAT

You don't have to start Phase 1 on a Monday, but I find this is the easiest way to stay organized. From the Master Food List for this phase, you will eat:

- Three carb-rich, moderate-protein, low-fat meals

- Two fruit snacks

Your day will look like this:

BREAKFAST	SNACK	LUNCH	SNACK	DINNER
Grain	Fruit	Grain	Fruit	Grain
Fruit		Protein		Protein
		Fruit		Veggie
		Veggie		

PHASE 1 EXERCISE

Do at least one day of vigorous cardio, like running, the elliptical trainer, or an upbeat aerobic-based exercise class during Phase 1. Cardio is perfectly suited for high-carb Phase 1.

In this phase, if you are a carb-lover, you get all the good stuff you love and crave—fruit and pasta, rice and crackers, toast and pretzels. These high-carb, moderate-protein, low-fat foods nourish the adrenals and soothe physiologic stress. I really want the body to fall in love with food during this phase, so it feels good and easy and fun to be in Phase 1.

Sweet fruits and whole grains stimulate the endorphins in the brain and flood the body with very easily accessible nutrients, making Phase 1 seductive and nurturing all at the same time.

Biologically, the goal of this phase is to really flood the body with nutrients, which stimulates the activity of the five major players in digestion and metabolism that we talked about earlier: the liver, the adrenals, the thyroid, the pituitary, and the tissues of the body. The adrenals are particularly nourished by the high but steady rate of natural-sugar delivery, making everything calm down and start to work better. The adrenals respond to blood sugar peaks and valleys by creating stress hormones that specialize in storing fat. But when blood sugar remains more stable (even if elevated at a healthy level), the adrenals calm down and begin to metabolize fat more efficiently. This balancing of the sugars is crucial in an individual who has become diabetic, insulin resistant, hypoglycemic, has had aggressive weight gain, or has elevated triglycerides.

Phase 1 foods are also designed to be rich in nutrients that stimulate the metabolism. Specifically, they are rich in B vitamins and vitamin C. The B vitamins are found in beans, meats, and whole grains, and they stimulate the thyroid, igniting the thermogenic (fat-burn) effect that revs up the metabolism. Those B vitamins are crucial in the metabolism of fats, proteins, and carbohydrates. Vitamin C in fruits like oranges and strawberries, as well as in vegetables like broccoli and sweet potatoes, helps the body convert glucose into energy, one of the primary goals of Phase 1. They help shuttle that glucose into the mitochondria—your cells' own little fat furnaces—to be broken down and converted to energy instead of being stored as fat. The abundant B vitamins you'll be getting during this phase also help support the adrenals in stimulating fat metabolism and lean muscle development.

Phase 1, **Unwind**, gently persuades your metabolism that it is no longer in an emergency situation. It's okay to actually digest the food you are eating again, to use the energy and nutrients from that food, rather than storing it as fat to guard against future starvation or nutritional deprivation. For the first two days, we are reteaching your body how to turn the food you eat into energy rather than storing it as fat. We're telling it, "Shh, shh, it's going to be okay." And with the foods you'll eat here, your body will believe it.

Your body starts to feel like everything really might be okay again. This is the first step in the three-step process.

It's the stimulation of digestive enzymes that helps accomplish this process in Phase 1. When you flood your body with so many nutrients and so much energy, it can actually start breaking down the foods you're consuming and releasing the nutrients embedded in these nutrient-dense foods. We want digestion to be as effortless as possible, which is why we keep protein moderate and fat very low. Fat and protein are harder to digest than carbohydrates like grains and fruits, so by keeping these low, the body is soothed and encouraged. Digestive enzymes release the vitamins and minerals and phytonutrients from the food you eat, and the metabolism begins to recover from its starvation state. Phase 1 foods are specifically designed to be easy on your body. You're ditching all those things that physically stress you, those metabolism crushers like wheat, dairy, and caffeine, that cause irritation or inflammation in the GI tract and can slow your bowels and create insulin resistance. Those things are all out of the game for now. Phase 1 will calm down your adrenal glands, reducing the release of stress hormones that are keeping you fat. Your blood sugar stabilizes and your body suddenly feels like it's out of the danger zone.

Phase 1 is kind to your body and kind to you. The sweeter tastes and comfort foods ease you, physically and also emotionally, into the plan. A lot of dieters haven't been able to touch these foods with a ten-foot pole for months, even years. It's time to normalize again. Phase 1 *feels normal,* not like a diet at all.

Low-carb dieters tend to panic when they see the list of foods for this first phase because they've been taught to believe carbs are bad. Carbs are *not* bad, food is not bad—if you choose healthy sources. Fruits, brown rice, oatmeal, alternative grains like quinoa and amaranth, lentils, beans—they are all good. The carbs you *won't* be eating during this phase are refined sugars, wheat, or corn. These carb sources are much harder on your body, and most people have ingested way too much of them over their lifetimes.

But if you're not a low-carb dieter and you're used to eating a lot of refined sugars and processed foods that don't require much digestive work, your body's going to have to gear up for the job, too. Foods high in refined sugar make the pancreas, adrenals, thyroid, liver, and gallbladder get lazy. It's like you've been plodding away on the elliptical trainer at a slow pace that barely distracts you from watching the *Today* show on the gym TV, and then you get a personal trainer who steps in and shows you a more efficient way to exercise. But this isn't boot camp. This is a kinder, gentler trainer who helps you condition in a way that doesn't exhaust you, but instead gives you more energy and stamina.

We're pampering and nourishing now, not abusing. We're breaking old patterns, not indulging them. The B vitamins in this phase will help modify a natural sense of panic your body may temporarily feel from being without habit-forming refined sugars and white flour.

What else can you expect during this phase? No more feelings of starvation! You won't be eating any refined sugar, juice, or dried fruit in this phase—that's making things *too* easy and allows the metabolism to get sluggish and lazy. But juicy apples and pears, pineapples and strawberries, watermelon and oranges? Fruit smoothies and spelt pretzels and brown rice pasta and oatmeal? Go for it!

In addition to the fruit and whole grains in Phase 1, you'll also be eating high-quality proteins like organic chicken, organic turkey, and even buffalo, as well as herbs and spices like parsley and cilantro that will help stimulate digestive enzymes, so you're getting plenty of protein your body can easily digest. Everything you eat will be nutrient-dense because nutrient-dense foods require a greater caloric expenditure from the body to extract their nutrients. This wakes up the body's organs and digestive enzymes and basically signals: *Hop to it, fellas, we've got some work to do!* My clients love this phase for all the wonderful comfort foods that don't make them feel like they are dieting. Another benefit of Phase 1 is that good carbs boost your mood, help you with crazy sugar cravings, and even ease you out of your caffeine funk, if you are (as I will strongly recommend) purging caffeine from your body during the next 28 days. These Phase 1 foods help head off that "crash" feeling. So does the frequency of eating—you'll be eating five, sometimes even six times per day, so get used to it!

GLYCEMIC—WHAT'S IT MEAN?

You've probably heard the word *glycemic* before reading this book, as in "glycemic index" or "low-glycemic foods" or "high-glycemic foods." It's trendy to talk about the glycemic index, but most people don't know exactly what it is. The way I always explain it to my clients is that it's the rate of sugar delivery of a food. Let's say you have a cup of orange juice and a cup of sliced oranges. Maybe both contain 23 grams of sugar, but the glycemic index, or GI, of the orange juice is higher than the GI of the orange slices because the body converts the sugar in the orange juice to sugar in the bloodstream much more quickly than it can convert the sugar in the orange slices. The fiber in the orange slices slows down the process; it's missing from the juice.

The problem with very high GI foods, like refined sugars taken out of their normal "package" (the orange, for example) and made into juice or cane sugar or maple syrup or any other sweetener, is that they are converted in the bloodstream *too* quickly. When the body gets too much sugar at once—in other words, more than it can use for energy and store in the muscles for quick energy—it starts shuttling that sugar directly into the fat cells.

Phase 1 uses high GI foods, but not super-high GI foods. That's why we don't have juice, dried fruit, any kind of refined sugar, or even the highest-sugar fruits, like bananas and grapes. Instead, we focus on fruits and fiber-rich whole grains to keep you in that sweet spot, where the body is getting plenty of sugar for energy, but not more than it can handle, so it doesn't store any more fat.

Calm, happy, and living in a land of plenty—that's what we're going for in Phase 1. We are sending your body the signal that everything it needs is readily available. We are extracting nutrients from food and feeding the adrenals, and happy, fed adrenals will set a body up for fat release. It is not in a state of famine. If you've been chronically dieting, your body will recognize this stage with a huge metaphorical sigh of relief.

Why will you lose weight in Phase 1? I like to illustrate what's happening in your body like this: Imagine that your best friend asks you to host her engagement party, at your house. She wants fancy hors d'oeuvres, a cake, party favors, decorations. You're already busy and you have no idea how you can handle it all, and you know you're either going to have to decline or stress yourself to the max. It's totally overwhelming.

This scenario is like you asking your body to lose weight when you're already stressed and nutrient-deprived. Your body may say, "I'm so sorry, but I can't accommodate that request." Or it's going to do what you want, but it's not going to be happy about it. You're not going to look or feel good. It's going to be hell.

But imagine, instead, that your friend asks you to host her engagement party, but she says, "I know you're busy, so I'm going to have a cleaning service come over and clean your house for you. I'm going to have the whole event catered, and I'll have a full staff come over to serve and clean up. Afterwards, I'll have a carpet-cleaning company come to clean your carpets." Now how would you feel about the task? Not so bad a prospect, right? In fact, it might even be fun! You're not used to getting that level of service, even when you aren't hosting a party! So what happens when the serving crew arrives, and somebody says, "Oh, no, we forgot the forks!" What are you going to do? You're going to be feeling so good, so energized, so *not* inconvenienced by it all, that you're going to skip into the kitchen with a big grin on your face and say, "Forks? No problem. I can provide forks."

This alternative scenario is like you asking your body to lose weight *while on Phase 1*. If you give your body the natural sugar, carbs, fiber, and protein it needs to function with ease and comfort, then your request for fat burning is going to be no big deal. So your body isn't getting fat during Phase 1? It's just like the forks. Your body is going to be happy to give over some fat to burn because it's so *not* inconvenienced by other dietary restrictions. It's got plenty of what it needs to feel good. Burn fat? No problem. Your body is getting the support it needs to handle the job, so the job becomes simple, joyful, and easy.

When you go on the Fast Metabolism Diet, you are asking the same thing of your body that you ask on a starvation diet, weight loss, but the terms are different—so different that it changes everything.

But Phase 1 isn't without rules. The one thing you won't be feeding your body during Phase 1 is very much fat. This is not the time for almonds and avocados. By delivering the carbs and proteins without the fat, we make the body start metabolizing its own fat stores to find the fat it needs. This is where the body's hard work comes in for Phase 1, a phase that feels easy to you but is actually pretty challenging for your body. We distract the body by flooding it with delicious carbs and protein, nourishing it while we also force it to go searching for fat. You'll start burning your own fat, not your muscle, because you won't need what the muscles contain. You're getting that from the food. While your body's having a natural-sugar-happy party, it barely notices that the fat burning has begun in earnest.

This is why we do Phase 1 first. We flood the body with nutrients and jump-start your system in a way that challenges your body while also feeling deliciously indulgent.

WHAT A DAY LOOKS LIKE—PHASE 1

In Phase 1, you are going to wake up in the morning and have breakfast within 30 minutes of waking. You will have a grain and a fruit, such as oatmeal and berries (no nuts or flax seeds, please—these are Phase 3 foods), or honeydew and a slice of spelt or brown rice bread. My assistant loves hot brown rice cereal with organic frozen peaches. I also have a client who puts oats in her fruit smoothie (find the recipe for her Oatmeal Fruit Smoothie on page 185).

Three hours later, you'll have a snack that consists of fruit. You might choose mangos or pineapples, tangerines or watermelon or strawberries.

Three hours later, lunch consists of a grain, a protein, a vegetable, and a fruit, all from your Phase 1 grocery list. You might choose a Chicken and Broccoli Bowl (page 191), or Turkey, White Bean, and Kale Soup (page 190), or turkey bacon with lettuce and tomato on sprouted-grain bread, along with peaches or grilled pineapples or a baked apple. And remember to use your leftovers. If you're on your second day of Phase 1, you can eat leftovers from dinner the night before.

For your afternoon snack, you get to have more fruit—maybe throw a tangerine or an apple in your bag, or slice and enjoy a juicy pear.

For dinner, you'll have a grain, a vegetable, and a protein. Maybe you'll enjoy filet mignon with broccoli and brown rice pasta, or turkey chili, or chicken and wild rice. Mmm, just telling you about it is making me hungry!

PHASE 1 SUPER SIMPLE CRASH STASH SNACKS

Apple

Orange

Frozen mango

Frozen pineapple

For more Phase 1 snacks, see the recipes in Chapter Eleven.

So for the next two days, we are reteaching your body how to turn the food you eat into energy rather than storing it as fat. You've been storing fat where you don't want to be storing fat, and we'll take care of that very soon, but this first step is to get your body to start actually burning the food you are actually consuming.

And that's Phase 1! It's only two days, and it's going to feel great. Just remember: fruit and grains, lean protein, and almost no fat. Those are the keys. Got it? Great!

Let's move on to Phase 2.

PHASE 2—UNLOCK FAT STORES
YOUR POCKET GUIDE

THE BASICS

This is the very high-protein, high-vegetable, low-carbohydrate, and low-fat phase.

High in foods that support liver function (so it can help cells release fat) such as:

Leafy greens	Onions
Broccoli	Garlic
Cabbage	Lemons

High in lean proteins such as:

Lean beef	Lean pork
Buffalo/bison	Tuna
White-meat chicken and turkey	Turkey bacon
Low-fat fish, like cod, flounder, and halibut	Nitrate-free jerky

Rich in alkalizing green, low-glycemic vegetables such as:

Kale	All kinds of lettuce
Mustard greens	Arugula
Collard greens	Watercress
Swiss chard	

High in carnitine-producing foods such as:

Beef	Cod
White-meat chicken	Asparagus

No fruit or grains

Low in fat

HOW TO EAT

If you started Phase 1 on Monday, then Phase 2 will always be on Wednesday and Thursday. From the Master Food List for this phase, you will eat:

- 3 high-protein, low-carb, low-fat meals
- 2 protein snacks

See the complete food list at the end of this chapter.

Your day will look like this:

BREAKFAST	SNACK	LUNCH	SNACK	DINNER
Protein	Protein	Protein	Protein	Protein
Veggie		Veggie		Veggie

PHASE 2 EXERCISE

Do at least one day of strength training (weight lifting) during Phase 2. Focus on lifting heavy weights with low reps. Lifting weights during Phase 2 will seriously increase your metabolic power, so go for it! If you aren't sure how to do it safely, see if someone at your local gym can guide you through the free weights, or take a class that uses weights, like Body Pump.

Phase 2 features foods that are completely different from the foods you ate during Phase 1—foods that push your metabolism to lay down muscle and scavenge fats. They are loaded with lean proteins that the body converts to amino acids that can be easily converted into muscle. The proteins mixed with the targeted vegetables make it virtually impossible to store any of the consumed foods as fat, and because you have just come off of Phase 1, where the adrenals have been soothed and the cortisol levels seduced into submission, your body is primed to release fat cells from the hips, butt, belly, and thighs. The amino acids are also the perfect food to stimulate the liver and vitalize the fat-shuttling mechanism in your body that begins to increase your metabolic rate. Not only are you burning your food for fuel but you are also beginning to burn your fat for fuel, so be diligent with your foods and pump that iron—your purposeful eating is beginning to take effect.

This phase is about an intensive altering of the body's structure converting stored fat to fuel to be transformed into muscle. It is so focused and intense that we only do it for two days. It is all about the muscle, and remember, muscle ravages calories (potential energy), so the more muscle you have, the more fat you'll burn. Sustaining and maintaining muscle takes energy, the constant contraction and relaxation of each and every muscle in your body requires fuel. The more muscle, the more fat you burn. On the contrary, have you ever seen your fat do anything but hang around on your belly?

The more muscle you build on the Fast Metabolism Diet, the more food you can consume down the road, and the higher your body will set its metabolic rate. The result of this high-protein, low-carb, low-fat phase is to rev up muscle and release stored fat. In Phase 1, you encouraged your body to calm down and actually start digesting the food you are eating rather than storing it. Now, you'll be eating specifically to absorb protein and release fat.

The foods in Phase 2, **Unlock**, allow for the mobilization of stored energy in the form of fat, so that you can actually burn it as fuel. The lean protein and large amount of vegetables in Phase 2 are the keys to this release. They "unlock" the stored fat, releasing it into the bloodstream. This preps your body for Phase 3, when it will actually focus on stimulating hormone production to burn quickly through all of the newly released fat. But you can't burn your fat cells until you unlock them for burning.

Are you seeing how this all begins to fit together? In Phase 1, you corrected the most urgent problem—encouraging your body to unwind and relax so it can start burning the food you eat again. Now, you're unlocking the fat. Finally, you'll burn it—but not until it's ready. Phase 2 gets that fat where it needs to be, so it is accessible as fuel.

To do this, you'll get to enjoy pork tenderloin and halibut, egg-white omelets and tuna, steaks and chicken, and all the green veggies you love, like broccoli and spinach, asparagus and mushrooms, celery and fennel and kale. And I'm not talking a half cup of this or that. I'm talking major vegetables. I'm talking 4 cups of broccoli, a mound of asparagus, a great big fistful of spinach. Go to town on those vegetables because they unlock the magical process of turning protein into beautiful muscle.

Focusing on lean protein and low-glycemic vegetables during Phase 2 promotes the retention and development of muscle, while we release body weight, primarily in the form of fat. Remember what I told you about how your body bypasses your fat and cannibalizes its own muscle for energy when you aren't providing it with enough nutrients? Phase 2 makes sure that doesn't happen anymore.

This phase is very low-glycemic. That means it doesn't contain foods that elevate your blood sugar very much. After all those yummy fruits and grains during the two Phase 1 days, now you're going in the opposite direction. The next two days are all about lean proteins like white-meat chicken and turkey, white fish and lean cuts of beef, lean pork, game meats like venison and elk, and egg whites. You're also going to get serious with low-glycemic, alkalizing vegetables—mostly the green ones, like cabbage and cucumbers, broccoli and kale, lettuce and spinach, and other non-starchy vegetables like mushrooms, red bell peppers, and onions.

Muscle is built from amino acids, which come from the breakdown of consumed protein. A nice, steady stream of easily digestible (meaning low-fat) protein will keep building muscle. This is so crucial in Phase 2.

The more muscle mass you have, the faster your metabolism will be. It's a simple equation: less muscle equals a slower metabolism. That's why we flood the body with proteins during Phase 2, and that's also why we push the carbohydrates so low. We want to encourage muscle building and fat burning, rather than burning sugar from carbohydrates, as we did in Phase 1. Remember: we want to confuse it to lose it!

Phase 2 also stimulates the liver in a different way, replenishing it with the nutrients and alkalizing effects of green vegetables. In Phase 2, we focus on amino acids, and specifically, on how they promote healthy liver function. The high-protein, low-glycemic foods in Phase 2 are liver foods. Your liver is responsible for over 600 metabolic functions, including converting every nutrient you consume into a bioactive form so it is available for your body to use. The liver is what stimulates your body to release fat cells from storage. It's essential to this process, so don't deviate from the Phase 2 food lists and maps! They are specifically designed to stimulate the liver by breaking down the proteins into amino acids and converting them into liver-supporting compounds like carnitine.

Earlier we briefly discussed carnitine. It is one of those powerhouse metabolism-stimulating nutrients that help the body release stored fat into the bloodstream so it can be metabolized for energy. It's the shuttle, or transport, compound that releases fat cells to be delivered directly to the fat-furnace mitochondria in the cells. Eighty to 90 percent of your metabolism action happens right there, in this teeny part of your cell. Eating the foods that stimulate this conversion from protein to amino acids to carnitine gives us ready access to those fat furnaces. When we get the fat to the furnace, it can burn.

Phase 2 foods stimulate the gallbladder, the guy that breaks down fats, and the pancreas, the guy that breaks down proteins (it also produces the insulin that regulates blood sugars so he was nurtured a lot in Phase 1). Phase 2 is also priming both these essential organs to produce the specific digestive enzymes they're going to need in Phase 3 for fat metabolism. See how this is a major metabolic workout and why all of this cross-training of your metabolism is going to allow you to use food to make you lose weight?

Phase 2 also floods the body with vitamin C, which tonifies and strengthens the adrenal glands that you just nourished in Phase 1. The stronger your adrenal glands, the less reactive they'll be in times of stress. Phase 2 helps stress-proof your body, strengthening your core physically, hormonally, and emotionally.

In addition, the bitter green vegetables you'll be eating provide a lot of nutrients for the thyroid, such as taurine and iodine, to facilitate the proper thyroid hormone production that we will be counting on for Phase 3. Also, because you are still minimizing fat intake, your body will continue foraging for body fat to burn.

During this phase, your body lays down the most amount of muscle mass, built with the high protein you're eating. But the high protein you're eating isn't the only thermogenic body builder—so are the alkalizing green vegetables you'll be eating so much of these two days.

Why are alkalizing vegetables so crucial? Because for healthy functioning, your body must maintain a certain pH level. That means the amount of acid in your bloodstream has to be kept within a certain range for life to continue and for your body to function well. This pH can be affected by what you eat. Some foods, like meat, tend to stimulate acid production, because it takes more acid to break down and digest meat. Diets that focus on large amounts of meat without the addition of a lot of alkalizing vegetables can cause the body to become too acidic, putting it into a state of keto-acidosis. During this state, you might hyper-mobilize fat, but at great expense. Many people dieting this way become carb resistant and prone to aggressive weight gain once they deviate from this way of eating. It is also hard on the kidneys, increases stress hormones, and increases systemic inflammation. Doing a high-protein diet without all the veggies also slows down your metabolism horrifically, putting you into an even worse state than you were to begin with. As soon as you go off this pure-protein diet, you'll gain 40 pounds. I've seen it happen over and over again. If you've been on a diet like this, your metabolism is likely to require some serious repair. If you were ever a body builder in a past life, you also understand the muscle-related dangers of the body from becoming too acidic—they get lactic acid buildup and they can't lay down muscle efficiently.

The magic of Phase 2 is that it combines high protein with a huge amount of green vegetables, and green veggies are alkalizing. The large volume of vegetables during Phase 2 is crucial in preventing the body from going into this unwanted state of acidity. These veggies also stimulate digestive enzymes that increase the rate of fat burn, like kindling for your fire. Most vegetables are alkalizing, but low-glycemic green vegetables tend to be the most alkalizing of all. That's why certain diets that promote green juices and green smoothies often advertise themselves as alkaline diets.

Green vegetables do wonderful things for you when you are upping your ingestion of meat protein, so shovel 'em in to keep your body's pH in check and everything running smoothly. Think of it this way: the protein is the log and the green vegetables are the kindling. It's hard to light a log, but add kindling and you'll have a crackling fire in no time. Put protein and alkalizing green vegetables together and your metabolism will ignite.

Your body is perfectly primed to digest all this protein now, specifically because we've already tickled your digestive enzymes during Phase 1, but the digestive enzymes stimulated by all the vegetables in Phase 2 will enhance this digestive effect even more dramatically. Now we can really push the envelope with protein, but because we still keep the fat low, your digestion is even more challenged than it was in Phase 1. Whew, what a metabolic workout! But remember, it is only for two days, then we will be on to the next phase of healing and repair.

We're building your body's capabilities back up gradually, with the help of all the phytonutrients in these low-glycemic vegetables. Green vegetables, in addition to being alkalizing, are rich in nitrogen, which is essential for muscle building. Nitrogen also helps the body break down all that protein into the amino acids that will be delivered to the muscles to promote muscle retention and development. All the protein you're eating will be easily incorporated into your body. Phase 2 literally transforms your body's composition, building muscle where you need it and torching fat where you don't, taking the raw materials and creating a beautiful temple called you.

My meat-loving clients really enjoy this phase, and former low-carbers are comfortable here, too. If you love a dinner of steak and salad, or pork loin and broccoli, or filet of sole with asparagus, you'll enjoy this phase. You probably won't even miss those carbs because you just had so many of them during Phase 1. And remember, Phase 2 only lasts for two days. Those two days will fly by when you think about how much fat you're **Unlock**ing and how much metabolism-firing muscle you're building.

WHAT A DAY LOOKS LIKE—PHASE 2

In Phase 2, you are going to wake up in the morning and have breakfast within 30 minutes of waking. You will have a lean protein and a veggie, such as an egg-white omelet with spinach or turkey bacon wrapped in lettuce leaves.

Two or three hours later, you'll have a protein snack. You can add green veggies to it if you like. You might choose buffalo jerky or roast beef with cucumber slices or a few pieces of nitrate-free deli chicken.

Lunch consists of another protein and vegetable. You might choose grilled chicken on salad with lettuce and lots of Phase 2 veggies, or Tuna Salad–Stuffed Red Pepper (page 201). And don't forget that you can also have leftovers from any Phase 2 dinner.

For your afternoon snack, you get to have more protein—maybe more jerky or three hard-boiled egg whites or tuna in celery.

For dinner, you'll have another protein and more veggies. Maybe you'll enjoy Broiled Halibut with Broccoli (page 209), chicken breast with asparagus, or Pepperoncini Pork Roast (page 212) with steamed spinach. If you aren't used to eating low-carb, Phase 2 may seem Spartan, but remember, it's only for two days and it's doing great things for you! Also, it might be easier than you think because low-carb meals tend to suppress the appetite, as long as you don't stay on them for too long.

PHASE 2 SUPER-SIMPLE CRASH STASH SNACKS

Turkey jerky

Canned tuna in water

Smoked salmon with cucumber

Hard-boiled egg whites

For more Phase 2 snacks, see the recipes in Chapter Eleven.

WHAT IF YOU DON'T LIKE LOW-CARB?

And if you don't love this stage? Phase 2 can feel difficult if you love your fruit, your starches, your morning oatmeal, but it's just for two days, and you're going to accomplish a lot. Everything you've fed your body in Phase 1 is nourishing your building efforts in Phase 2. Like I said, it's only two days. You don't have to be over-the-moon about Phase 2. That's fine. We're repairing the metabolism here, not sending you to an amusement park. If it really irritates you to eat like this, go take it out on some really heavy weights. Leave it all at the gym and feel the burn as you sculpt your body.

Think of it this way: if you have to go to physical therapy for an injury, you probably love the massage part, but you might hate the 4,000 daily toe flexes. But both are essential for your recovery. Some parts are tough, but it's all part of the rehabilitation, so if you find yourself whining, here's what I have to say to you: I am proud of you for existing outside of your comfort zone. You're more than fine. You are doing the work that needs to be done to heal. So keep it up.

Besides, it's time for Phase 3, and you're going to *love* it there.

PHASE 3: UNLEASH THE BURN—HORMONES, HEART, AND HEAT
YOUR POCKET GUIDE

THE BASICS

This is the high healthy–fat, moderate-carbohydrate, moderate-protein, low-glycemic fruit phase.

High in healthy fats such as:

Nuts and seeds	Olives
Avocados	Olive oil
Coconuts	

Higher-fat proteins in moderate amounts such as:

Salmon	Hemp seeds
Sesame and almond butter	Hummus

Lower-glycemic fruits such as:

Blackberries	Cranberries
Blueberries	Grapefruit
Raspberries	Lemons and limes

Lower-glycemic vegetables such as:

Artichokes	Eggplant
Asparagus	Spinach
Beans	Seaweed
Cauliflower	Sweet potatoes
Leafy greens	

Moderate amounts of unrefined carbohydrates such as:

Barley	Quinoa
Wild rice	Sprouted-grain bread
Oatmeal	Quinoa pasta

Thyroid-stimulating foods such as:

Seaweed	Shrimp
Coconut oil	Lobster

Foods rich in inositol and choline such as:

Legumes, like black beans, chick- peas, kidney beans, and lentils	Nuts and seeds
	Brussels sprouts
Beef and chicken liver	

HOW TO EAT

If you started Phase 1 on Monday, then Phase 3 will always be on Friday, Saturday, and Sunday. From the Master Food List for this phase, you will eat:

- 3 meals

- 2 healthy-fat snacks

See the complete food list at the end of this chapter.

BREAKFAST	SNACK	LUNCH	SNACK	DINNER
Fruit	Healthy Fat	Fat/Protein	Healthy Fat	Fat/Protein
Fat/Protein	Veggie	Veggie	Veggie	Veggie
Grain		Fruit		Grain/Starch
Veggie				

PHASE 3 EXERCISE

Do at least one day of stress-reducing activity like yoga, or deep breathing, or enjoy a massage during Phase 3. Yes, massage counts! It's not an "activity" per se, but it increases blood flow to the fatty areas of your body, reduces cortisol, and does the work we want for you during this phase.

Phase 3 is exciting, delectable, and powerful—the phase where we **Unleash** the full power of a stoked metabolism and where we focus on what I like to call the "thermogenic three": hormones, heart, and heat. These three are responsible for cranking up the metabolic heat in the body and really boosting the burn. In this phase, after four days of eating low fat, you're going to bring the fat back for the next three days. Your body is perfectly primed for it now—your digestive enzymes are firing, your muscles are pumped up, your body is richly fed with nutrient-dense foods, and now, just when you really need it, heart-healthy fats come flooding in, triggering your body's fat-for-fuel mechanisms. You begin burning the fat you're eating, as well as all the fat you unlocked in Phase 2. Phase 3 is a high-fat, moderate-carbohydrate, moderate-protein, low-glycemic fruit phase.

In Phase 3, you're really going to start seeing some changes. This is the phase that flattens your belly and irons out your cellulite—that makes you look different, that makes people ask, "Hey, have you lost weight?" (Of course, you'll be able to reply, "Why, yes. Yes I have.") This phase is all about heat and it's the stage of the plan that makes you look *hot!*

Phase 3 is different from the first two phases in that it is three days long instead of two. It might just be the most critical phase of Fast Metabolism, and yet it couldn't exist without Phase 1 and Phase 2 laying the groundwork.

All week, you've kept your fat intake very low, as you suffused your body with nutrients from targeted carbohydrate sources, loads of green vegetables, and quality protein. In the absence of dietary fat and plenty of nutrition, your body has been burning fat. And burning fat. And building muscle. But by the fifth day of the week, your body is beginning to get suspicious. *Wait a minute*, it thinks. *There hasn't been much fat coming in. Maybe we'd better start storing some?*

Au contraire! says Phase 3. *You don't have to worry one bit. Here's some fat for you—lots of delicious, wonderful, healthy dietary fat!*

Although this phase is high in fat, it's not high in just any old fat. No fried foods or hunks of cheese, please. Instead, Phase 3 focuses on healthy fats like avocados, nuts, seeds, as well as olive, sesame seed, and grapeseed oils.

Eat this way and here's what happens. In Phase 2, the nutrients from all those green vegetables helped restore and replenish the very organs and glands that are responsible for major fat burning. The gallbladder, in particular, primed by the pancreas, now knows how to torch fat like nobody's business. Just like you need to have money to make money, you need to eat fat to burn fat, and that's exactly what happens in Phase 3.

The energy released from breaking down fat cells is truly profound. It's money hidden in the vault under your bed beneath the concrete, but the Fast Metabolism Diet is your pickax, and when you break through, there are phenomenal health benefits, not only in disease prevention but in how you feel right now. People complain and whine and moan about the fat on their bellies, their hips, under their chins. I say, good for you! You've got something to burn, and all the benefits to reap.

SCIENCE-GEEK MOMENT

Don't neglect your vegetable serving at breakfast during Phase 3! This is very important. Vegetables contain cellulose, and when you consume a lot of cellulose, your body creates a lot of proteolytic enzymes in order to break everything down into usable and digestible components. When we eat a lot of fat, we want to make sure it is also broken down and converted to energy. You can't have the fat consumption and the fat release without this breakdown if you want the fat to get out of your body. This phase isn't complete without the breakdown, and that breakdown is facilitated by vegetables.

Remember, like Phase 1, Phase 3 can be deceptive because it feels so good. But you are still doing a lot of internal work. You're happy to do it because you've got all those feel-good hormones coursing through your brain, making you feel satiated and content, but it's still work to scavenge all that surface fat and digest it. It requires a lot of energy, and energy requires food. I've told you before that calories in *do not* equal calories out, and this is true nowhere more than in Phase 3, but this won't work if you aren't eating your vegetables. Even for breakfast.

When you start providing your body with all that beautiful, rich, good fat, after all the work your body has been doing to find fat to metabolize in your own body, now it gets a rest. You flood your body with dietary fat, and your body goes, "Ahhhh, there it is." And then it starts burning its own fat, right along with the fat you are eating! The dietary fat that is so easy to break down helps release a flood of fat-melting enzymes from the gallbladder that then go postal on your own fat stores, rooting them out and tossing them in the metaphorical furnace. Ironically, eating fat *after* not eating it for a few days makes you start burning fat like crazy. This is a classic example of why by **Unwind**ing your stress hormones, **Unlock**ing stored fat, and **Unleash**ing fat-burning hormones, you keep the metabolism guessing. This is exactly why the "confuse it to lose it" method is so effective.

This phase is intense and powerful. The influx of good, healthy dietary fats feeds your brain and your sex drive, your thyroid, and also your adrenal glands. Everything starts humming along like a well-oiled machine. Because fat contains more energy than carbs or protein, you may notice a surge of energy during Phase 3. Blood flow increases and your metabolism starts to burn even hotter. In Phase 3, two very interesting things are happening at once: the intensity of the fat burn and the wonderful, relaxing effect of having enough fat intake.

Just like yoga lowers stress hormones, so does Phase 3 by providing the nutrients the body needs to generate anti-stress hormones.

All this fat burning and hormone production is a big job, though. It feels good, but it's also intense. Part of the intensity of this phase is due to your body's purging a lot of toxins stored in your fat that have now been released. So it will be extremely important to drink a lot of water especially now, and keep your bowels moving. Even consider taking a sauna during Phase 3 to help sweat out some of the toxins. It's so important and vital to keep everything moving out. This toxin release contributes to your new thinner, tighter look because, when the toxins come out, so does the swelling and inflammation and even some of those lumpy bumpy spots (aka, cellulite). But if you don't release the toxins and excess fat, they're just going to get reabsorbed into your body. You'll take fat from your right hip and put it on your left hip. You'll take dimples off your belly and put them on your butt. That's not what we're going for here. We want to flush them away. We want them gone.

Envision that thick yellow fat hanging out in your bloodstream (you released it from your fat cells in Phase 2) just starting to evaporate. Phase 3's hormones help convert that fat into water-soluble substances that you can easily break down in the mitochondria for energy and that can also be easily excreted through the sweat, urine, and blood. It's all melting away, baby, and you're looking good!

If the toxin concentration is too dense, your kidneys will send a red alert out to the hypothalamus, adrenals, pituitary, and thyroid to slow things down again. It's the last thing we want to do during the release process, so it's crucial to have enough water on board. Water helps dilute the toxins, so the excretory process doesn't cause as much stress.

But you'll hardly notice the physiological intensity of Phase 3 (especially with sufficient water intake) because you'll be too busy enjoying the yummy healthy-fat foods you love, like avocados and salmon, almond butter and walnuts. You can cook with sesame oil, drizzle olive oil on your salads, and dunk your veggies in hummus or guacamole. It's all so rich and decadent and delicious—and so good for you, too!

During Phase 3, you'll focus on targeted metabolism-stimulating nutrients that work fast to kick the fat out of the body. For example, Phase 3 foods are rich in inositol and choline, key cofactors that metabolize fat and keep it from getting blocked in the liver. These nutrients, found in rich amounts in egg yolks and raw nuts and seeds, are like goalies for the fat that gets released. They block the fat from being reabsorbed and help knock it out of the body, so it doesn't get stored somewhere else.

We also eat fatty fish in this phase, which lowers cortisol levels and helps promote healthy hormone balance in the thyroid and adrenal glands. Avocado is another Phase 3 star, and it contains a unique starch called manahexolose, which helps balance blood sugar, reduce insulin resistance, and really light the metabolism on fire. There is also another nutrient found in raw nuts and seeds that actually slows gastric emptying. We call these "feel-full fats." The longer it takes to empty the food from your stomach, the better chance that meal will stimulate the hypothalamus and pituitary to signal your body that you are full and satisfied. Phase 3 foods also produce endorphins, those feel-good hormones that make you feel like you've had enough and you don't need to eat anymore.

The fats in olive oil cause a dramatic increase in fat oxidation or fat burning in the body, especially stimulating the burn of brown fat, which helps your body to burn more and more fat as fuel. In fact, from the first moment you put that buttery avocado or creamy almond butter in your mouth and start chewing, your pituitary will begin releasing hormones that help break down fat.

Phase 3 also contains a lot of lysine. Lysine is an amino acid that contributes to that shrink-wrap effect you're getting during Phase 3, where your cellulite flattens and your muscles look more defined. This is an old aggie trick. We supplement horses or cattle with lysine before a show to accentuate their muscle definition. Lysine can work for you in the same way, visibly making you look better. Lysine specifically helps scavenge cellulite and surface fat. One of my clients told me that she lost 30 pounds on another diet and people said, "Did you get a haircut?" But when she lost her first 9 pounds on this diet, people said, "You look amazing, how much weight have you lost!" It's the lysine effect.

You'll get a lot of lysine to help eliminate that blanket of fat covering all the fantastic muscles you've been building, and you'll get it in Phase 3 foods, especially in nuts like hazelnuts and almonds, seeds like sesame and pumpkin seeds, nut butters and pastes (especially the sesame paste and tahini), coconut, egg yolk, and avocado.

FAST METABOLISM FACT

Every phase of the Fast Metabolism Diet nurtures the heart in some way. The cardiologists at one of the clinics I consult with think I'm a miracle worker. But you and I know the truth—it's just the three phases at work! You see, the heart is made of smooth muscle tissue, just like your biceps and triceps. Like any other muscle, heart function is dependent on the muscle's ability to relax and contract; so in Phase 2, with all that protein, you helped to build and heal your heart muscle. In Phase 3, you're providing the heart-healthy omega-3 fatty acids (the ones in fish and walnuts and olive oil) that keep everything moving slickly and smoothly through the heart. When you get back to Phase 1 in the second, third, and fourth weeks, you'll notice a marked increase in your ability to do cardio easily. We only do cardiovascular activity for two out of the seven days in each week, but when you're on the Fast Metabolism Diet, that's all you'll need. Every phase helps the heart, so at the end of the 28 days, you'll not only be thinner, stronger, and healthier, you'll be heart-healthier, too.

Although decadent-feeling fats are high in Phase 3, don't let that fool you into thinking you can eat *everything* during these three days. Phase 3 is a lower-glycemic phase, for a very important reason. Phase 3 is *not* just Phase 1 plus fat. In Phase 1, we had a lot of high natural-sugar foods that are easy to digest. Fat is the hardest thing to break down, requiring the most energy from the body, so if we elevate the sugar intake too much during Phase 3, the body will default to burning that sugar and it won't burn the fat. Low-glycemic foods are essential in Phase 3 for this reason. You've got to sprinkle in enough carbohydrates to keep your energy going, but not so much that you override the fat-burning effect.

That's the reason behind why this is not the time to eat a lot of fruit and starch. You'll notice when you review the meal maps that you get a grain and a fruit with breakfast, a fruit with lunch, and an optional grain with dinner, but both snacks don't contain fruit or grain and lunch does not include any grain. It's very important to stick to this for Phase 3, so the fat-burning magic can happen. The carbs in Phase 3 are just to tease fat metabolism.

Although this phase feels great, it's also intense for the body, even though you're loving the food, so that's why we do it for three days, and then we stop. That's it. We take a break and carb you up again when you circle back around to Phase 1 and begin the next week of the plan. You might really enjoy the benefits of this phase, but don't stay here longer than three days because we have more work to do.

Thank that extra padding on your butt and thighs and belly because it's helping your body remember how it's really supposed to work. Your fat is a teaching tool! And as you burn it, your body learns, and remembers, so that after the diet is over, you'll keep burning the fat you eat and using the fat you store for fuel—your metabolism will work just the way it was intended to work. And you won't store more fat than you need to store anymore.

WHAT A DAY LOOKS LIKE—PHASE 3

In Phase 3, you are going to have breakfast within 30 minutes of waking. You will have a healthy fat, a protein, fruit, grain, and a veggie, all from the Phase 3 food list (see page 80). An example might be an omelet (use the whole egg during this phase) with spinach, tomatoes, and mushrooms on sprouted-grain toast, or a bowl of oatmeal with raw almonds, peaches, and almond milk plus some cucumber slices or celery with lime juice and salt.

Celery and Almond Butter

Raw nuts and seeds

Avocado

Hummus and Cucumber

Creamy Guacamole

For more Phase 3 snacks, see the recipes in Chapter Eleven.

It's easy to include vegetables when you are eating eggs, but even if you are eating oatmeal or toast, you must add the vegetable. This will help keep the fat-release shuttle open and also enhance the healthy digestion of fats. There are so many enzymes in vegetables that help this process along, and you need them! You want all the little fat cells in your butt and thighs to jump on that enzyme wagon to go make hormones and muscles and energy.

For a snack you might have ¼ cup hummus with veggies, and lunch could be an Avocado and Turkey Lettuce Wrap (page 223), or a big green salad with chicken breast, and lots of Phase 3 veggies dressed in olive oil or the Phase 3 dressing (page 222). You could even heat up some leftovers from a Phase 3 dinner—just remember to ditch the grain. Then dinner might be Shrimp Stir-fry (page 231) or Avocado Chili (page 229).

Sometimes, my clients get confused about how best to include fat in their meals. I say, "liberally!" For example, I had a client ask, "If I'm making a stir-fry, can I also put avocados in my salad?" My simple answer, Yes! Because you are only including healthy fats, I want you to use them liberally. Have the stir-fry, the avocados, even the olive-oil-based salad dressing. Dip your veggies in creamy hummus or rich guacamole. Slather your celery with almond butter. It's all good. And it's only for three days. The fat you are eating is amping up the thermogenic process, so have at it! As long as you stick to the Phase 3 food list at the end of this chapter and meal maps, you're golden.

Next up . . . the rules of the road.

PHASE 1 FOOD LIST
(select organic whenever possible)

VEGETABLES AND SALAD GREENS (FRESH, CANNED, OR FROZEN)

- Arrowroot
- Arugula
- Bamboo shoots
- Beans: green, yellow (wax), French
- Beets
- Broccoli florets
- Cabbage, all types
- Carrots
- Celery, including tops
- Cucumbers
- Eggplant
- Green chiles
- Green onions
- Jicama
- Kale
- Leeks
- Lettuce (any except iceberg)
- Mixed greens
- Mushrooms
- Onions, red and yellow
- Parsnips
- Peas: snap, snow
- Peppers: bell, pepperoncini
- Pumpkin
- Rutabaga
- Spinach
- Spirulina
- Sprouts
- Sweet potatoes/yams
- Tomatoes
- Turnips
- Zucchini and winter or yellow summer squash

FRUITS (FRESH OR FROZEN)

- Apples
- Apricots
- Asian pears
- Berries: blackberries, blueberries, mulberries, raspberries
- Cantaloupe
- Cherries
- Figs
- Grapefruit
- Guava
- Honeydew melon
- Kiwis
- Kumquats
- Lemons
- Limes
- Loganberries
- Mangos
- Oranges
- Papaya
- Peaches
- Pears
- Pineapples
- Pomegranates
- Strawberries
- Tangerines
- Watermelon

ANIMAL PROTEIN

- Beef: filet, lean ground
- Buffalo meat, ground
- Chicken: skinless, boneless white meat
- Corned beef
- Deli meats, nitrate-free: turkey, chicken, roast beef
- Game: partridge, pheasant
- Guinea fowl
- Haddock fillet
- Halibut: fillet, steak
- Pollock fillet
- Pork: tenderloin
- Sardines, packed in water
- Sausages, nitrate-free: turkey, chicken

Sole fillet

Tuna, solid white, packed in water

Turkey: breast meat, lean ground

Turkey bacon, nitrate-free

VEGETABLE PROTEIN

Black-eyed peas

Chana dal/lentils

Chickpeas/ garbanzo beans

Dried or canned beans: adzuki, black, butter, great northern, kidney, lima, navy, pinto, white

Fava beans, fresh or canned

BROTHS, HERBS, SPICES, AND CONDIMENTS

Brewer's yeast

Broths: beef, chicken, vegetable*

Dried herbs: all types

Fresh herbs: all types

Garlic, fresh

Ginger, fresh

Horseradish, prepared

Ketchup, no sugar added, no corn syrup

Noncaffeinated herbal teas or Pero

Mustard: prepared, dry

Natural seasonings: Bragg Liquid Aminos, coconut amino acids, tamari

Pickles, no sugar added

Salsa

Seasonings: black and white peppers, chili powder, cinnamon, crushed red pepper flakes, cumin, curry powder, nutmeg, onion salt, raw cacao powder, sea salt, Simply Organic seasoning

Sweeteners: Stevia, Xylitol (birch or hardwood only)

Tomato paste

Vanilla or peppermint extract

Vinegar: any type

GRAINS AND STARCHES

Amaranth

Arrowroot

Barley

Brown rice: rice, cereal, crackers, flour, pasta, tortillas

Brown rice cheese or milk

Buckwheat

Kamut: bagels

Millet

Nut flours

Oats: steel-cut

Quinoa

Rice milk, plain

Spelt: pasta, pretzels, tortillas

Sprouted-grain: bagels, bread, tortillas

Tapioca

Teff

Triticale

Wild rice

HEALTHY FATS

None for this phase

*Note: All broths, if possible, should be free of additives and preservatives.

PHASE 2 FOOD LIST
(select organic whenever possible)

VEGETABLES AND SALAD GREENS (FRESH, CANNED, OR FROZEN)

Arrowroot

Arugula

Asparagus

Beans: green, yellow (wax), French (string)

Broccoli florets

Cabbage, all types

Celery

Collard greens

Cucumbers, any type

Endive

Fennel

Green chiles, jalapeños

Green onions

Jicama

Kale

Leeks

Lettuce (any except iceberg)

Mixed greens

Mushrooms

Mustard greens

Onions, red and yellow

Peppers: bell, pepperoncini

Rhubarb

Shallots

Spinach

Spirulina

Swiss chard

Watercress

FRUITS (FRESH OR FROZEN)

Lemons

Limes

ANIMAL PROTEIN

Beef, all lean cuts: filet, tenderloin, strip, sirloin, shell steak, London broil, round steak, rump roast, stew meat, lean ground

Buffalo meat

Chicken: boneless, skinless white meat

Cod/scrod fillet

Corned beef

Deli meats, nitrate-free: roast beef, chicken, turkey

Dory fish fillet

Eggs, whites only

Flounder fillet

Game: venison, ostrich, elk

Halibut fillet

Jerky, nitrate-free: beef, buffalo, turkey, elk, ostrich

Lamb, lean cuts

Oysters, packed in water

Pork: loin roast, tenderloin

Salmon: nitrate-free smoked

Sardines, packed in water

Sole fillet

Tuna, packed in water

Turkey: breast steaks, lean ground

Turkey bacon, nitrate-free

VEGETABLE PROTEIN AND STARCHES

None this phase

BROTHS, HERBS, SPICES, AND CONDIMENTS

Brewer's yeast

Broths: beef, chicken, vegetable*

Dried herbs: all types

Fresh herbs: all types

Garlic, fresh, powdered

Ginger, fresh

Horseradish, prepared

Mustard: prepared, dry

Noncaffeinated herbal teas or Pero

Natural seasonings: Bragg Liquid Aminos, coconut amino acids, tamari

Pickles, no sugar added

Seasonings: black and white peppers, cayenne, chili powder, chili paste, chipotle, cinnamon, crushed red pepper flakes, cumin, curry powder, raw cacao powder, nutmeg, onion salt, sea salt, Simply Organic seasoning

Sweeteners: Stevia, Xylitol

(birch or hardwood only)

Tabasco

Vanilla or peppermint extract

Vinegar: any type (except rice)

GRAINS
None this phase

HEALTHY FATS
None this phase

PHASE 3 FOOD LIST
(select organic whenever possible)

VEGETABLES AND SALAD GREENS (FRESH, CANNED, OR FROZEN)

Arrowroot

Artichokes

Arugula

Asparagus

Avocados

Bean sprouts

Beans: green, yellow (wax),

French (string)

Beets: greens, roots

Bok choy

Broccoli

Brussels sprouts

Cabbage, all types

Carrots

Cauliflower florets

Celery

Chicory (curly endive)

Collard greens

Cucumbers

Eggplant

Endive

Fennel

Green chiles

Green onions

Hearts of palm

Jicama

Kale

Kohlrabi

*Note: All broths, if possible, should be free of additives and preservatives.

Leeks

Lettuce (any except iceberg)

Mixed greens

Mushrooms

Okra

Olives, any type

Onions

Peppers: bell, pepperoncini

Radishes

Rhubarb

Seaweed

Spinach

Spirulina

Sprouts

Sweet potatoes/ yams

Tomatoes, fresh and canned: round, plum, cherry

Watercress

Zucchini and winter or yellow summer squash

FRUITS (FRESH OR FROZEN)

Blackberries

Blueberries

Cherries

Cranberries

Grapefruit

Lemons

Limes

Peaches

Plums

Prickly pears

Raspberries

Rhubarb

ANIMAL PROTEIN

Beef: filet, steaks, lean ground

Buffalo meat

Calamari

Chicken: boneless, skinless dark or white meat, ground

Clams

Corned beef

Crab, lump meat

Deli meats, nitrate-free: turkey, chicken, roast beef

Eggs, whole

Game: pheasant

Halibut fillet

Herring

Lamb

Liver

Lobster meat

Oysters

Pork: chops, loin roast

Rabbit

Salmon, fresh, frozen, or nitrate-free smoked

Sardines, packed in olive oil

Sausage, nitrate-free: chicken, turkey

Scallops

Sea bass fillet

Shrimp

Skate

Trout

Tuna, packed in water or oil

Turkey

Turkey bacon, nitrate-free

VEGETABLE PROTEIN

Almond milk, unsweetened, almond cheese, almond flour

Cashew milk

Chickpeas/ garbanzo beans

Dried (or canned) beans: adzuki, black, butter, Great Northern, cannellini, kidney, pinto, white, lima, navy

Hemp milk, unsweetened

Lentils

GRAINS

Barley, black or white

Oats: steel-cut, old-fashioned

Quinoa

Sprouted-grain: bread, bagels, tortillas

Wild rice

BROTHS, HERBS, SPICES, CONDIMENTS, AND SUPPLEMENTS

Brewer's yeast

Broths: beef, chicken, vegetable*

Carob chips

Dried herbs: all types

Fresh herbs: all types

Garlic, fresh

Ginger, fresh

Horseradish, prepared

Ketchup, no sugar added, no corn syrup

Mustard, prepared, dry

Natural seasonings: Bragg Liquid Aminos, coconut amino acids, tamari

Noncaffeinated herbal teas or Pero

Pickles, no sugar added

Salsa

Seasonings: black and white peppers, cinnamon, chili powder, crushed red pepper flakes, cumin, curry powder, onion salt, raw cacao powder, turmeric, sea salt, Simply Organic seasoning

Sweeteners: Stevia, Xylitol (birch or hardwood only)

Tomato paste

Tomato sauce, no sugar added

Vanilla or peppermint extract

Vinegar: any type (except rice)

HEALTHY FATS

Avocados

Coconut, coconut milk, cream, water

Hummus

Mayonnaise, safflower

Nuts, raw: almonds, cashews, hazelnuts, pecans, pine nuts, pistachios, walnuts

Nut/seed butters and pastes, raw

Oils: coconut, grapeseed, olive, sesame, toasted sesame (Asian)

Seeds, raw: flax, hemp, pumpkin, sesame, sunflower

Tahini

*Note: All broths, if possible, should be free of additives and preservatives.

CHAPTER FOUR

Fast Metabolism Rules: The Do's and Don'ts

N̲ow that we know why and how the diet works, it's time to make it start working for you. In this chapter, I'm going to lay down the rules. I'm going to tell you exactly what you need to eat (and what few foods are off limits) for the next 28 days to make the weight loss happen. The next 28 days aren't business as usual. This is your intense repair session. If you want it to work, you have to follow the rules. No arguing, no deviating. For the next four weeks, these rules are nonnegotiable.

The rules are easy, straightforward. They aren't scary. I want you to *confuse it to lose it*, but I don't want to confuse *you*.

I want to make it fun. So here's a rule you're going to like: You have to eat. In fact, the #1 rule on the Fast Metabolism Diet is that you have to eat five times, every single day. That's 35 times per week. And no cheating by skipping meals! You're going to eat, and you're going to eat a lot. And you're *still* going to lose weight.

But none of it will happen if you don't eat according to the strategically designed plan I've created. The rules are crucial if you want the diet to work.

Let's make friends with the word *DIET*—not the word *diet*, but the acronym D.I.E.T. It stands for: Did I Eat Today? As in:

Did I eat every three to four hours today?

Did I eat within a half hour of waking today?

Did I eat according to my phase today?

Did I eat enough complex carbohydrates (Phase 1), lean protein and green vegetables (Phase 2), or healthy fats (Phase 3) today?

Did I Eat Today? That's your new meaning for the word *DIET*. I don't want you ever to associate the word *DIET* with deprivation and starvation again. The new *DIET* is all about eating.

If you're going to do this, you have to realize that you're going to have to change some of what you've been doing, even if you don't always like it. I won't make you eat something you're allergic to or morally opposed to or really hate, but the rules allow for those differences. If you broke your leg, would you tell the doctor, "I'm sorry, Doc, but I can't wear that cast. It doesn't look good on me. And I don't really feel like using the crutches." No, of course not. If it's broken, you wear the cast. Following the doctor's rules is a medical necessity; following my rules of repair is a metabolic necessity!

Read them carefully. Then read them again. They apply to all the phases and give specifics on living each phase that are crucial. While they are not "forever" rules, you might feel so healthy and full of energy for the next 28 days that you *want* to stick with some of them—or maybe even all of them—for the rest of your life. Remember, none of us is caffeine or artificial-sweetener deficient. Even if you don't buy into the theory that some of the things we are eliminating during the next four weeks have a negative impact on your health, I can assure you that they are not at the top of my list of things I would use to get you healthy.

FAST METABOLISM DO'S AND DON'TS

THE DO'S

RULE #1: YOU MUST EAT FIVE TIMES PER DAY, 35 TIMES PER WEEK.

That's three meals and two snacks every day. The good news is that you *get* to eat 35 times per week, so when I tell you that you won't be starving or missing fruits or carbs or fats or protein, I mean it.

You may not skip any meals or snacks. This is crucial to repair the metabolism. It's nonnegotiable. I don't care if you don't think you're hungry. You have to eat.

RULE #2: YOU MUST EAT EVERY THREE TO FOUR HOURS, EXCEPT WHEN YOU'RE SLEEPING.

This may mean even more eating than five times a day! If you stay up late or go for more than three or four hours without eating, you must add an additional phase-specific snack. For example, if you *finish* eating dinner at 7:00 and you don't go to bed until 11:00 or 12:00, you must have a third phase-specific snack three to four hours after you finish dinner. If you're worried about how to fit all this eating into your busy schedule, don't be. My clients are all exceptionally busy people, just like you, and they find the time to eat every three to four hours. The key is to time it to your individual schedule. The following chart gives you some examples of how to do this if you keep relatively average hours, if you're an early riser, a late riser, or someone who works the night shift. The last row is for you to fill in your own typical schedule:

	WAKE UP	BREAKFAST	SNACK	LUNCH	SNACK	DINNER
AVERAGE SCHEDULE	7:00 A.M.	7:30 A.M.	10:00 A.M.	1:00 P.M.	4:00 P.M.	7:00 P.M. (finish at 8:00 P.M.)
EARLY RISER	5:00 A.M.	5:30 A.M.	8:30 A.M.	11:00 A.M.	2:00 P.M.	5:00 P.M.
LATE RISER	9:00 A.M.	9:30 A.M.	11:30 A.M.	2:30 P.M.	5:00 P.M.	8:00 P.M.
NIGHT SHIFT	2:00 A.M.	2:30 A.M.	5:30 A.M.	8:30 A.M.	11:30 A.M.	2:30 P.M. (finish at 3:00 P.M.)
YOU						

RULE #3: YOU MUST EAT WITHIN 30 MINUTES OF WAKING. EVERY DAY.

Don't wait to have breakfast. If you are dashing out the door and you don't have time to sit down for a full meal, you can have your morning snack first and your breakfast when you get to work. But you must eat something within that first 30 minutes so your body doesn't have to run on fumes. Also, please *don't exercise* before you put something in your stomach. I like to tell my clients, "Don't fast and then go fast." You might think you're burning more fat this way, but in reality it is one of the worst things you can do to your metabolism.

RULE #4: YOU MUST STAY ON THE PLAN FOR THE FULL 28 DAYS.

The plan lasts for 28 days for a reason: to follow the natural circadian rhythm of the body. Individual weeks can be repeated again and again for additional weight loss, but the initial commitment has to be for the full four weeks to get true repair in all phases of the body. It's like sweeping off the patio. Your first run-through you don't get everything, so you have to go back through and catch what you didn't catch the last time.

RULE #5: YOU MUST STICK TO THE FOODS ALLOWED IN YOUR PHASE.

You must do this *religiously*. If you are in Phase 1 and it's not on the food or meal map for Phase 1 days, don't eat it. The same goes for all three phases.

There are also foods left off the lists and maps, and that's not a mistake or a typo. These things are intentionally left off. In the Don'ts section after, I'll explain why certain foods are left off. For now, know that if it's not on any of the lists or the maps, you're not going to eat it for the next 28 days.

RULE #6: YOU MUST FOLLOW THE PHASES *IN ORDER*.

That means two days of Phase 1 followed by two days of Phase 2 followed by three days of Phase 3. And it is easiest to follow if you start the plan on a Monday.

As you know from the last chapter, each of the phases is designed with a particular goal (**Unwind**—calming the body to facilitate the absorption of nutrients from food, **Unlock**—building muscle and releasing stored fat, and **Unleash**—burning fat) and in a specific order for a reason.

RULE #7: YOU MUST DRINK HALF YOUR BODY WEIGHT IN OUNCES OF WATER EVERY DAY.

For example, if you weigh 200 pounds, that's 100 fluid ounces of water every day. If you weigh 180 pounds, that's 90 fluid ounces of water each day. Once you've met that required amount, you can have noncaffeinated herbal tea, or make lemonade with fresh lemons and limes sweetened with a natural sweetener like Stevia or Xylitol (but *not* with sugar, honey, maple syrup, or agave nectar). However, tea and lemonade do not count toward your required water ounces.

Limit any naturally sweetened drink to no more than two per day. I don't want your taste buds to get too accustomed to the taste of sweet beverages, even if they don't have any glycemic value. And remember—the water comes first!

RULE #8: EAT ORGANIC WHENEVER POSSIBLE.

I understand that at times organic food can be more expensive, and not everybody believes that organic food is better or healthier. I'm not going to argue that point either way, but it's a fact that any synthetic chemical products you put into the body—including additives, preservatives, pesticides, insecticides, and hormones—have to be processed through the liver. This monopolizes time and energy that could be used to repair your metabolism. Remember, I'm trying to be greedy with the liver's energy here. So eat as cleanly as possible. Also, try to keep your environment as clean as possible. This is not a time to paint the inside of your house or recarpet. These kinds of environmental chemicals have to be processed through your liver, too, and that will keep your liver distracted from the job we want it to do: burn fat.

There are so many delicious raw nut butters out there that you won't even miss the absence of peanut butter on the Fast Metabolism Diet. I love peanut butter, but because it is one of the dirtiest products out there (it grows in the ground and contains so many agricultural chemicals) and because it is not typically sold raw (way too moldy), it's not a part of your life for the next 28 days. If you have it again after the 28 days are over, choose organic peanut butter without added sweetener, but for now, stick to raw almond, cashew, hazelnut, sesame, and yummy raw sunflower butter. You won't even miss the peanuts.

RULE #9: MEATS MUST BE NITRATE-FREE.

Nitrates are substances that are typically added to cured meat products— like bacon, turkey bacon, sausages, jerky, and packaged deli meats (including the stuff behind the meat counter)—to impede bacterial growth, so the food doesn't spoil as quickly. Because nitrates do this by slowing down the breakdown of fat in the meat, they also slow down the breakdown of fat in the body, just when we're trying to do the opposite: melt the fat faster!

Instead, eat meat that is cured and preserved naturally, with foods like celery juice and sea salt. These are perfectly safe and easy to find. Most supermarkets and all natural foods stores carry them, and several major food brands now make them, too. If you aren't sure about a product, look at the ingredients label for words like "nitrate-free" and "naturally cured," or ask the butcher if the meat is preserved with nitrates. Local organic meat producers also often have nitrate-free options. Just remember that these meats don't last quite as long, so keep them frozen until the day before you are ready to eat.

RULE #10: EXERCISE ACCORDING TO YOUR PHASE.

The Fast Metabolism Diet is about food, but it isn't *only* about food.

PHASE 1: Do at least one day of vigorous cardio, like running, the elliptical trainer, or an upbeat aerobic-based exercise class.

PHASE 2: Do at least one day of strength-training with weights.

PHASE 3: Do at least one day of stress-reducing activity like yoga or deep breathing, or enjoy a massage. It's not an "activity" per se, but it increases blood flow to the fatty areas of your body, reduces cortisol, and does the work we want for you during this phase.

THE DON'TS

If you've already flipped ahead to check out the recipes, meal maps, and food lists, you might have noticed that a few things you're used to eating aren't on any of the lists. But I have very good reasons for why I'm temporarily taking them off the menu. These foods make it *harder,* if not impossible, to reset and repair the metabolism.

We've come together for a common goal, so let's stick with it. You won't be giving up these foods forever. For now, though, they're out. But so you're totally with me on this, let's talk about why.

RULE #1: NO WHEAT.

Wheat is a billion-dollar agricultural business. To increase the crop yield, and thus profits, farmers have hybridized wheat to make it sturdy enough to withstand the most extreme weather conditions (remember, I'm an aggie and I took many courses on this). As a result, it has become not just indestructible in the field but also nearly indestructible in your body—in other words, it's very hard for your body to digest and extract its nutrients.

Think about it this way: If wheat can withstand a hailstorm and bug infestations, what chance has your body got to break it down? Among other things, it creates inflammation, gas, bloating , water retention, and fatigue. Going wheat-free might sound intimidating, but I promise you won't miss it. You can eat so many better, healthier carbs on this diet, like brown and wild rice, barley and quinoa, or breads and pastas made with sprouted grains or spelt.

You may not be used to eating these grains, but you can find any of them (or any other foods on the food list, for that matter) at any well-stocked supermarket or health food store. *Wheat in a sprouted form* is the *exception to the no-wheat rule* and sprouted wheat or wheat-free baked products like bread, bagels, and tortillas are usually found in the freezer section (so they stay fresh). Enlist your store manager if you would like more options. They are often willing to order a product for you if they know you're going to buy it.

RULE #2: NO CORN.

Corn is one of your metabolism's worst enemies. That's because farmers, as with wheat, have drastically modified corn to increase yields. But there's another reason. Vegetarians might want to skip this next sentence: when farmers want to increase the marbling (or white tissue fat for flavoring) in beef to increase the grade of the meat, they feed the cows lots of corn right before slaughter. In other words, corn equals quick fat. They also feed corn to horses before a show when they've dropped too much weight. Essentially, the corn kernel has become, through the miracles of genetic engineering, a big reservoir for sugar that ramps up white fat production. If you eat lots of corn, you might bring more money if sold at market, but you will not be a metabolic marvel.

I have many actor clients, and occasionally one will ask me to help him or her *gain* weight for a part in a movie when they need to look chubby. Corn is one of my best tricks. If you want to look pregnant or have a poochy belly, round cheeks, and plump arms, eat corn. If you want a fast metabolism, do not.

RULE #3: NO DAIRY.

"But I just looooove cheeeeese!" my clients whine. I hear you. Cheese tastes good. But cheeses, and all other dairy products, have a sugar-fat-protein ratio that wreaks havoc when repairing your metabolism. The rate of sugar delivery from the lactose (milk sugar) in dairy is way too fast, and the animal-based fat is too high.

I know what you seasoned dieters are thinking: what about low-fat cottage cheese and Greek yogurt? These foods do have health benefits, like protein, and they can have a place in your life . . . but not for the next 28 days. Contrary to what you might think, the worst form of dairy is any nonorganic, *fat-free* variety. When it comes to dairy, repeat after me, "If it says free, it's not for me." Fat-free dairy aggressively slows fat metabolism.

The other problem with dairy is that it stimulates the sex hormones in metabolism-stalling ways. Even organic products contain amino acid ratios that alter the balance of the sex hormones. I use full-fat dairy in my fertility diet, and encourage many women trying to get pregnant to drink organic whole milk. But it isn't appropriate on this program.

Don't worry; I won't leave you without any options. You can use unsweetened rice milk during Phase 1, and you can use unsweetened almond milk or unsweetened coconut milk during Phase 3. No milks of any kind are allowed during Phase 2, but it's only two days out of the week. You can handle it.

RULE #4: NO SOY.

Sorry, soy lovers. It's true that non-GMO tofu, edamame, and tempeh can be healthy foods, especially if you don't eat animal protein, but not when you are trying to heal your metabolism. Soy is estrogenic in nature, meaning it contains plant estrogens that are close to the estrogens your own body manufactures, and I know no other substance more perfectly suited to increase belly fat. Plus, most soy is genetically modified, which makes it harder for your body to break down.

In conventional cattle raising, soy is used as filler in livestock feed to increase the protein ratios cheaply, much the way fast-food restaurants sometimes add soy protein to their hamburgers. The estrogenic effect of soy also causes rapid weight gain: good for livestock bad for you.

I had a client, an actor, who was extremely fit, thin, and healthy. He needed to look like a chronic alcoholic—like he'd been drinking for a week straight, his whole life going out of control. I had 14 days to make him look the part. No problem! I knew just what to do. I fed him a bunch of soy, and in 14 days he looked like he'd been hitting it hard and heavy for years. Soy slows the metabolism, and it doesn't have a place in your life, at least not for the next 28 days. (Although if you never ate it again, I wouldn't be upset.)

And don't worry, vegetarians—there are plenty of other high-protein, meat-free foods you can eat on the Fast Metabolism Diet. All the meal maps in this book come with vegetarian options.

There are two exceptions to the no-soy rule: tamari and Bragg Liquid Aminos. That's because these are both extracts from a fermented soy product that doesn't contain the same estrogenic or bloating factor.

RULE #5: NO REFINED SUGAR.

Refined sugar is a very concentrated source of quick energy, and when the body has too much, when it becomes too readily available, the body has to work extremely hard just to maintain a stable, normal blood sugar level so you stay conscious and on your feet and alive. This becomes almost impossible in the presence of too much refined sugar because it's delivered into the bloodstream so rapidly and readily. To get rid of it, the body quickly shuttles it away to the fat cells, where it won't ramp up the blood sugar any further. It's a survival mechanism. So when you eat refined sugar, you are basically mainlining the stuff right into your fat cells.

Just 2 teaspoons of refined sugar can inhibit your weight loss for three to four days. Say you go out to a party and have just one soda or a piece of cake. Say good-bye to weight loss until next week. Even worse, you'll crave more sugar, and you'll want it *bad.* The most difficult time to avoid sugar is the next few days after eating sugar. There are many animal studies suggesting that sugar is as addictive to the brain and the body as cocaine.

Refined sugar also has a suppressive effect on your immune system. *Just 2 teaspoons of refined sugar will cut your T-cell count* (the white blood cells that are instrumental in keeping your immune system strong and functioning) *by 50 percent for two full hours after eating,* leaving you more vulnerable to infection and illness.

You might also be interested to know that refined sugar is highly impure. Many refined sugars are combined with a glycoprotein, which stimulates sugar to come through the gut wall even faster. What's more, and vegetarians should take note, they get that glycoprotein from pig's blood or bone char. The animal ingredients used in the process don't have to be disclosed, but they are there nonetheless. Yuck. Just get off the stuff . . . at least for the next 28 days.

RULE #6: NO CAFFEINE.

It's important to understand how much caffeine stresses your adrenal glands. Your adrenal glands are very important in regulating blood sugar, keeping your cortisol (stress hormone) levels steady, and regulating epinephrine and norepinephrine, the so-called fight-or-flight hormones. The adrenals also help regulate aldosterone, which controls fat metabolism, and regulate sugar storage and muscle development.

Caffeine pushes the body past its healthy state of energy, constantly stealing from your reserves, leaving you depleted and without resources for when you really need energy. Yes, I realize that coffee and caffeine have a reputation for decreasing appetite and contributing to weight loss, but the reality is that they only do this for people who are on an extremely low-carbohydrate, low-calorie diet—the kind of diet you'd better stay on forever if you want to achieve your weight loss this way because the minute you start eating normally again, you'll gain it all back, and more. Those who want to be able to live their lives and eat food are best off ditching the caffeine habit for the next 28 days . . . and maybe even forever.

Also, you should know that decaffeinated coffee is not truly caffeine free. Depending on the brand, it can still contain 13 to 37 percent of the caffeine of regular coffee. If you absolutely cannot see giving up coffee right now, your best bet is organic decaffeinated coffee. Just know that you are still getting a dose of adrenal-stressing caffeine.

And if you're going to push my buttons and insist on your morning coffee, you *must* eat before you drink it. If you ingest coffee with no food on board, your body will begin to pull sugar from your muscles in order to sustain the adrenal hormones being stimulated by the caffeine. Caffeine before breakfast is a metabolism-killer, and that includes noncoffee choices like black tea, green tea, and white tea.

The bottom line is that nobody is caffeine deficient. This is not a mineral required for your body. You may beg to differ, but you should know that ingesting caffeine is a fabulous way to screw up the metabolism.

I know this is hard. Caffeine is emotionally and physiologically addictive, and the withdrawal can be tough. But the good news is that after about three or four days of harsh symptoms, it'll be over. No more afternoon slump. No more obsessive need for a buzz. It's an incredible feeling to escape the caffeine monkey on your back.

Some of the tricks I use for helping people deal with caffeine withdrawal are:

- Cinnamon added to your morning smoothie

- Feverfew, an herb that can help with withdrawal headaches

- Gingko biloba, which is vaso-dilating and can also help with those headaches

- Patience. Just keep reminding yourself that in a few short days, you're going to wake up feeling like a million bucks.

RULE #7: NO ALCOHOL.

I know. You like your glass of wine, or your margarita, or whatever. I would never tell you that you can never have another drink. But here's the bottom line: Alcohol has to be processed through the liver. Again, that means it's also monopolizing a major organ that we're trying to heal. Telling you to avoid it is not a judgment about alcohol. It's not about the empty calories. It's about the metabolism.

Beyond the toll it takes on your liver, there are even more reasons to avoid alcohol for the next 28 days. Alcohol is very high in sugar, in that it converts to sugar rapidly in the bloodstream. That's exactly what we're trying *not* to do. I'll tell you how to incorporate alcohol safely into your Fast Metabolism life in Chapter Ten. For the next four weeks, though, your weight loss will happen more quickly and your metabolism will heat up more effectively if you stick to club soda with lemon or lime.

RULE #8: NO DRIED FRUIT OR FRUIT JUICES.

Raisins, dried cranberries, dried apricots—these can be good snacks once in a while. But not during this process. The sugar concentration is too high and the fiber is too easy to break down. When you eat dried fruit, or drink fruit juice, just as with the refined sugars we discussed earlier, the sugar in these foods gets delivered too rapidly into your bloodstream. This forces your body to store the excess in fat cells. Juice in particular increases the rate of sugar delivery because, while you might get the same grams of sugar from an orange as you would get from orange juice, the fiber in the whole orange slows down the rate of sugar delivery into the bloodstream. You can have your raisins in your oatmeal and your occasional small glass of orange juice again. Just not for the next four weeks.

RULE #9: NO ARTIFICIAL SWEETENERS AND RULE #10, NO FAT-FREE, "DIET" FOODS.

I always tell my clients, "If it's fake, take a break." If it says "Diet Something" or "Zero-Calorie Something" or "Fat-Free Something," put it back and step away from the shelf. No frozen diet dinners, no packaged junk food. No prepackaged 100-calorie snacks.

Convenience is not a bad thing, and many companies are creating healthy quick alternatives to "on the go" foods. But on this diet you'll be making your own prepackaged snacks and frozen dinners from real food, or finding fresh, real-food alternatives in delis and restaurants. It's easy and convenient and delicious, and you can do it.

And please, throw away the pink, yellow, and blue fake sugar packets. They are like poison for your body and your metabolism. If you must use a sweetener, use natural ones like Truvia, Stevia, or Xylitol instead.

And there you have it.

THE SECRET LIFE OF FOOD ALLERGIES

Ironically, the foods you crave the most may be the foods to which your body is most intolerant. When I was a child, I used to crave plain butter, and I would eat it right off the stick. Gross, right? But I couldn't help myself. I also suffered from eczema. I didn't know then that I was craving fat because my body needed it. Now I know that I need good fats, but I'm allergic to dairy. When I dropped the dairy, my skin cleared right up.

What's your weakness, your secret craving?

Sometimes, I ask my clients, "Let's say I have a magic wand and I can make your favorite or most craved food into the healthiest food on earth. What would you want me to use it on?" They admit that they are closet carb junkies or have intense cravings for sugar, chocolate, or cheese. That's when I gently suggest that maybe these are the exact foods they need to trim or eliminate from their diets, at least for a while.

THE RULES

These rules are simple and easier to follow than you may think. And if you need further incentive, know that following them makes you feel amazing. Many of my clients have loved how they felt so much that they incorporated these rules into their permanent lifestyles and never looked back. If you remember nothing else, remember this: eat five times a day, and only the foods on the list for your phase.

THE RULES AT A GLANCE

THE DO'S

Rule #1: You must eat five times a day. That's three meals and two snacks per day. No skipping.

Rule #2: You must eat every three to four hours, except when you're sleeping.

Rule #3: You must eat within 30 minutes of waking. Every day.

Rule #4: You must stay on the plan for the full 28 days.

Rule #5: You must stick to the foods allowed on your phase. Religiously. I repeat: only eat from the food list for your phase.

Rule #6: You must follow the phases in order.

Rule #7: You must drink half your body weight in fluid ounces of water every day.

Rule #8: Eat organic whenever possible.

Rule #9: Meat choices must be nitrate-free.

Rule #10: You must exercise three times per week, according to your phase.

Rule #1: No wheat.

Rule #2: No corn.

Rule #3: No dairy.

Rule #4: No soy.

Rule #5: No refined sugar.

Rule #6: No caffeine.

Rule #7: No alcohol.

Rule #8: No dried fruit or fruit juices.

Rule #9: No artificial sweeteners.

Rule #10: No fat-free "diet foods."

And above all, remember to think back to the acronym DIET: Did I Eat Today?

CHAPTER FIVE

Looking at Your Life: Making It Work for You

I've been pretty bossy with you. It's been my way or the highway. I had good reason—you need tough love at a time like this. But just in case you were beginning to think that I wasn't going to let you have your way about *anything,* this chapter will convince you otherwise. In fact, I *want* you to customize the Fast Metabolism Diet so it fits *your* life. It's your body, it's your food, it's your health, and it's your diet. You have to follow my rules—I'm not budging on that—but you can also shape the Fast Metabolism Diet to your individual circumstances, so you can actually do it successfully in your real life, in the real world.

I had a client once who came into my office, and even before he sat down, he started lecturing me: "Okay, I'm going to do this diet thing. And I'm willing to hear you out, but you should know that I can't eat this, and I can't eat that, and I can't eat this . . ."

"Whoa, wait a minute," I said, holding up my hand. "Sit down. Let's talk about this. Together we'll work out what you can eat and what you can't eat. What you are and aren't willing to do. Then we'll come to a compromise we can both live with, and I'll spit in my hand and you'll spit in your hand and we'll shake on it. Okay?"

There are so many variables that go into successful weight loss, and if you don't consider these, you set yourself up for failure. I want my plan to become *our* plan. I want us to customize this together so we can negotiate a deal that will not compromise your individuality, but also won't compromise your successful weight loss.

Clients come into my office all the time almost in a state of panic. They know they're about to "start a diet," and they get themselves all psyched out for what they think the reality of that diet is going to be. Sometimes they say things to me like, "I know this is going to be hell," or "I know this is really going to suck," or "I realize this is going to be the hardest thing I have ever done." Or they're more fatalistic, saying things like, "Well, I can't lose weight, but I'll try," or "I bet I'm going to be the one client that this diet doesn't work for," or "If I just lose five pounds, I'll still be grateful."

These moments break my heart. I know from my very long history with people trying to lose weight how difficult and painful it can be, and how often all the hard-won weight comes back.

But I promise this is going to be different. Yes, I have a strict program that I insist you follow. Plenty of aspects of the Fast Metabolism Diet are nonnegotiable. But this diet isn't painful. And there are plenty of negotiable, customizable aspects of Fast Metabolism. You can make it yours, not some prison sentence someone has imposed on you for your own supposed good.

I *want* to know what you like. What foods you love. I want to know, with no judgment, the good, bad, and ugly of your eating past. What are your obsessions? Mine are sour cream, butter, ice cream, avocados, and mayonnaise (obviously I like my rich, creamy foods!). I hate hard candies, but I love chilies and soups. I can eat pineapple until my lips fall off, but apples aren't my favorite.

I'm also an idealist. Every Monday morning, I start strong—but then all hell breaks loose at one of my clinics, or at one of the kids' schools. Or I have to jump on a plane or sit down for an interview. Or I have to interview a new chef and taste a boatload of food. So I plan for the worst and I have a Crash Stash snack in every car and office, and even in the front of my suitcase. I restock it every time I get home. But my weeks are always a challenge, so I try to make sure that my food isn't.

WHO ARE YOU?

What about you? What foods do you find hard to resist? Which ones aren't your favorites? Are you a picky eater, or will you eat anything? And how does your week usually play out? When do you tend to succeed, and where do you tend to make mistakes?

This is the "think about your life" chapter. The "let's spit in our hands and shake" chapter. I'm going to help you look at all the ways your life might not necessarily conform to a generic version of this diet, and then I'm going to help you make it work for you, the way I've made it work for hundreds of others.

Deal?

CHECK-IN TIME

Before you can customize the Fast Metabolism Diet effectively, you're going to have to get real about exactly who you are, what you do, what you like, and what you are probably not willing to do.

How much weight do you want to lose?

When do you get up in the morning?

Do you like to eat breakfast right away, or not until you get to work?

Do you have to cook for a family, or is it just you, eating whatever and whenever you want?

Do you avoid the kitchen at all costs, or are you constantly planning what to cook next?

Are you a vegetarian?

Do you have to eat gluten-free?

Are you an exercise fanatic, or has it been a while since you last hit the gym?

It's time to check in with yourself. Think about your habits and what happens when you have gone on diets before.

Do you love routine or hate it?

Does your job require an atypical schedule?

Are you a carb fanatic or a big meat eater?

Do you get hungriest in the afternoon, or at night?

Do you usually eat on purpose, or do you find yourself eating when you didn't intend to eat?

A lot of these questions are easy to answer if you do a simple exercise for me. I would like you to write in a diet diary for the next three days, to get a handle on the reality of your life, the timing of your days, and how we can fit Fast Metabolism into your schedule.

Here is an example of how you might make a diet diary. In addition to first answering the above questions, include every single bite you put in your mouth for three days. Think about whether it was an intentional meal or snack, or "accidental" noshing. Remember that honesty is the best policy here. We want to look at your reality so we can see any potential stumbling blocks and prevent disasters at all cost. You're doing this so the diet will *work*. So please: full disclosure.

ONE FULL DAY OF FOOD					
TIME	WHAT I ATE	MEAL OR SNACK?	PLANNED OR NOT?	HOW I FELT BEFORE	HOW I FELT AFTER

After you've collected three days' worth of this valuable information, take a good, hard, analytic look at the data. Do you tend to eat at the same times every day, or are your eating habits random? Do you get up early or sleep late? Do you rush out the door? Will it be tough to eat breakfast within 30 minutes of waking? Do you stay up late or eat dinner late? Are there foods you know you can't have on the Fast Metabolism Diet that you eat frequently? Are there foods on the diet you like but don't eat very much, that you might enjoy eating more of?

Compare your diet diary to the diet rules in Chapter Four, and see which ones might be a challenge for you. What can you realistically live with, and what has to be modified? Where are you going to have to compromise—cheese? sugar? And where are you going to feel like you're getting away with something great—avocados? almond butter?

Now let's break it down so we can make it all work for you.

YOUR DAILY SCHEDULE

The first thing to consider is your schedule. If you work outside the home and have a strict schedule, it will likely determine when and how you eat. For example, maybe you can't get up and have a good breakfast within 30 minutes of waking because you have to rush to the office, and you usually eat something there. No problem. As long as you eat *something* within the first 30 minutes of waking, you're still following the rules. Just switch your morning snack and your breakfast. Have an apple as you're getting ready for work, or a hard-boiled egg on the train. Once you get to work, make your phase-specific meal: your oatmeal or toast, eggs or turkey wrap, or celery with almond butter. You'll also need to think about which food choices will work when you aren't at home. If your office has a kitchen, great. If not, will you need to pack a breakfast the night before?

If you work the night shift, your schedule will be different. As long as you are eating within 30 minutes of waking, and every three to four hours after that, it doesn't matter what time of day you begin, whether that's 6:00 A.M., 6:00 P.M., or any other time.

Your work schedule or other aspects of your life may also impact when you have dinner. If you tend to eat dinner very late, you may need to have an afternoon and an evening snack before dinner to be sure you are eating every three to four hours.

Your daily schedule can also impact what day you start the diet. Although I generally recommend starting on Monday so you are in Phase 3 on the weekend, when the food choices are a little more liberal, this doesn't work for everyone. I have one client who has date night with her husband every Wednesday night. For her, it works best to start on Saturday. Saturday and Sunday are her carb-rich, sugar-rich Phase 1 days; this melds best with the way she eats on the weekends with her family. Monday and Tuesday are family dinner nights, so she cooks meat and vegetables for everyone, and finds it easy to adhere to Phase 2. On date night, she is in Phase 3, so she can go out for Mexican food and enjoy guacamole, or Middle Eastern food and enjoy hummus, or she can have salmon sashimi at a sushi restaurant. Thursday and Friday are her remaining fun Phase 3 days, and then by Saturday, she's ready for Phase 1 again.

Think about your own schedule in these terms—are there particular days when it would definitely be easier to be in a particular phase every week? Plan your start date based on that. Any schedule can work with the rules, especially if you always have Crash Stash snacks (see page 181) in your purse or desk. This is crucial. You can make the Fast Metabolism Diet work with your life, as long as you plan ahead.

YOUR PORTIONS

Every recipe in this book includes a portion size, but how much weight you have to lose also influences your portions. If you have a lot of weight to lose, it's going to take more food (not less!) to keep your metabolism roaring.

To figure out your portion sizes, first determine your goal weight. I'm not going to tell you what it is. You already know exactly how much you want to weigh and what weight makes you comfortable. Take what that number is, and compare it to your current weight, then look at the chart that follows to determine your portion sizes while you are on Fast Metabolism.

How much do you want to weigh? I'm asking you, not telling you, because you already know. It's a number that is completely unique and individual to *you*. It's the weight that makes you happy, and it has nothing to do with the weight that will make someone else happy.

I've had clients who weighed 250 pounds, and they knew they would be happy and comfortable at 180 pounds. Other clients feel best at 150 pounds, or 130 pounds. Your goal is to be able to feel and eat like a "normal person." No chart can tell you what that means for you.

I never recommend going by weight charts or the BMI. I hate the BMI! I just can't bring myself to recommend it to my clients. I'm not going to put any weight charts in this book because chronic dieters already have a number in their heads. When you reach it, you might decide to set a new goal. But for now, decide what you want to weigh, and write that number here:

My current goal weight is:

_____

IF YOU HAVE 20 POUNDS OR FEWER TO LOSE: Go by the basic portions listed below, and the portions included in the recipes in this book.

IF YOU HAVE 20-40 POUNDS TO LOSE: Add a half portion. For example, if a portion of chili is 2 cups, and you want to lose 30 or 40 pounds, then you would have 3 cups of chili.

IF YOUR LONG-TERM GOAL IS TO LOSE MORE THAN 40 POUNDS: A lot of clients come to me with these weight-loss goals, but I tell them, let's work at this 40 pounds at a time. So, that means you will be eating as if you want to lose only 40 pounds (i.e., the 3 cups of chili), with one exception: I require that you double your veggie portion. So if the suggested portion for someone trying to lose 40 pounds is 2 cups of spinach, I want you to eat 4 cups of spinach so we keep our eye on the long-term goal and use that food as the catalyst for continued weight loss.

LONG-TERM WEIGHT LOSS GOAL: 20 POUNDS

Food	Phase 1	Phase 2	Phase 3
Meat	4 ounces	4 ounces (2 ounces for snack)	4 ounces (2 ounces for snack)
Fish	6 ounces	6 ounces (3 ounces for snack)	6 ounces (3 ounces for snack)
Legumes/beans	½ cup	none	½ cup
Cooked grains: rice, pasta, quinoa	1 cup	none	½ cup
Crackers or pretzels	1 ounce	none	0.5 ounces
Bread, bagels, tortillas	1 slice bread, ½ bagel, 1 tortilla	none	1 slice bread, ½ bagel, 1 tortilla
Oats	½ cup uncooked, 1 cup cooked	none	¼ cup uncooked, ½ cup cooked
Fruit	1 cup or 1 piece	1 cup or 1 piece (lemons and limes only in this phase)	1 cup or 1 piece
Vegetables and salad greens	unlimited	unlimited	unlimited
Oils	none	none	3 tablespoons
Hummus	none	none	⅓ cup
Guacamole	none	none	⅓ cup
Avocado	none	none	½ avocado
Raw nuts	none	none	¼ cup
Raw nut and seed butters	none	none	2 tablespoons
Dressings	2-4 tablespoons	2-4 tablespoons	2-4 tablespoons
Smoothies	1 12-oz glass	1 12-oz glass	1 12-oz glass
Herbs	unlimited	unlimited	unlimited
Spices	unlimited	unlimited	unlimited
Broths	unlimited	unlimited	unlimited
Condiments	unlimited	unlimited	unlimited

LONG-TERM WEIGHT LOSS GOAL: 20-40 POUNDS

Food	Phase 1	Phase 2	Phase 3
Meat	6 ounces	6 ounces (3 ounces for snack)	6 ounces (3 ounces for snack)
Fish	9 ounces	9 ounces (4.5 ounces for snack)	9 ounces (4.5 ounces for snack)
Legumes/beans	¾ cup	none	¾ cup
Cooked grains: rice, pasta, quinoa	1½ cups	none	¾ cup
Crackers or pretzels	1.5 ounces	none	.75 ounces
Bread, bagels, tortillas	1 slice bread, ½ bagel, 1 tortilla	none	1 slice bread, ½ bagel, 1 tortilla
Oats	¾ cup uncooked, 1½ cup cooked	none	¾ cup cooked
Fruit	1½ cups or 1½ pieces	1½ cups or 1½ pieces	1½ cups or 1½ pieces
Vegetables and salad greens	unlimited	unlimited	unlimited
Oils	none	none	4½ tablespoons
Hummus	none	none	⅓ cup
Guacamole	none	none	½ cup
Avocado	none	none	¾ avocado
Raw nuts	none	none	⅜ cup
Raw nut and seed butters	none	none	3 tablespoons
Dressings	3-6 tablespoons	3-6 tablespoons	3-6 tablespoons
Smoothies	1 16-oz glass	1 16-oz glass	1 16-oz glass
Herbs	unlimited	unlimited	unlimited
Spices	unlimited	unlimited	unlimited
Broths	unlimited	unlimited	unlimited
Condiments	unlimited	unlimited	unlimited

LONG-TERM WEIGHT LOSS GOAL: MORE THAN 40 POUNDS

Food	Phase 1	Phase 2	Phase 3
Meat	6 ounces	6 ounces (3 ounces for snack)	6 ounces (3 ounces for snack)
Fish	9 ounces	9 ounces (4.5 ounces for snack)	9 ounces (4.5 ounces for snack)
Legumes/beans	¾ cup	¾ cup	¾ cup
Cooked grains: rice, pasta, quinoa	1½ cups	none	¾ cup
Crackers or pretzels	1.5 ounces	none	.75 ounces
Bread, bagels, tortillas	1 slice bread, ½ bagel, 1 tortilla	none	1 slice bread, ½ bagel, 1 tortilla
Oats	1½ cup cooked	none	¾ cup cooked
Fruit	1½ cups or 1½ pieces	1½ cups or 1½ pieces	1½ cups or 1½ pieces
Vegetables and salad greens	unlimited, but double my suggested portions	unlimited, but double my suggested portions	unlimited, but double my suggested portions
Oils	none	none	4½ tablespoons
Hummus	none	none	⅓ cup
Guacamole	none	none	½ cup
Avocado	none	none	¾ avocado
Raw nuts	none	none	⅜ cup
Raw nut and seed butters	none	none	3 tablespoons
Dressings	3-6 tablespoons	3-6 tablespoons	3-6 tablespoons
Smoothies	1 16-oz glass	1 16-oz glass	1 16-oz glass
Herbs	unlimited	unlimited	unlimited
Spices	unlimited	unlimited	unlimited
Broths	unlimited	unlimited	unlimited
Condiments	unlimited	unlimited	unlimited

And take note that vegetables are unlimited for everyone but, if your long term goal is to lose more than 40 pounds, you need to eat at double the recommended portion of veggies with each meals and snack. Still, no matter how much you have to lose, you can eat as many vegetables as you want. When it comes to vegetables, the more the merrier. They contain all those important enzymes and phytochemicals that encourage fat metabolism, so have at it.

When I tell people the portion sizes for the Fast Metabolism Diet, they tend to get nervous, especially if they have been on extremely calorie-restricted diets in the past. I have to keep reminding them that it takes energy to lose weight, and energy comes from food. So don't be afraid of these portions. This is your medicine. This is your fuel. As long as it's phase-specific, and you eat according to the meal map, the food you are eating will increase your metabolism so much that your body will combust all that food and more. Remember, starvation diets conserve fat. Diets that include eating enough real food *burn fat*.

COOKING FAT-FREE

In Phase 1 and Phase 2, when I can't use oils for cooking, I like to use organic vegetable broth to stir-fry vegetables and cook eggs and lemon and lime instead of oil for baking and broiling.

WHERE YOU ARE NOW

A lot of my clients are more likely to know their goal weights than to know their inches, but I like to take baseline measurements before my clients begin the Fast Metabolism Diet because measurements are much more about what you are building structurally than a number on a scale. This is why I'm not a fan of the BMI system of monitoring weight. You can weigh what looks like normal but not have a healthy body composition— for instance, you might have too much belly fat, even if the rest of you looks thin. Or, you can have a healthy distribution of weight even if you are above the "normal" range on the BMI chart.

That's why I suggest taking your measurements now, and recording them here. Take four:

Your hips at the widest part: _____ inches

Your waist at the belly button: _____ inches

The widest part of one thigh: _____ inches

The widest part of your upper arm: _____ inches

As you go through the 28 days of the Fast Metabolism Diet, monitor changes in these measurements, which I think are more exciting than any changes on the scale.

YOUR PERSONAL DEAL-BREAKERS

If you have dietary restrictions, the Fast Metabolism Diet can look challenging. What if you are vegetarian, or vegan, or you must eat gluten-free? No problem! There are so many options on this diet that you can easily adapt it to your dietary deal-breakers. Let's talk about each one individually:

VEGETARIAN

Any of the phases can easily be adapted to a vegetarian diet, especially if you are willing to eat eggs and fish while you are on the Fast Metabolism Diet. (I know that fish isn't technically vegetarian, but there are those who will make an exception and maybe you are one of them.) If not, though, for any Phase 1 and Phase 3 recipes that include meat, you can substitute ½ cup cooked legumes, like lentils, black beans, white beans, or any other phase-specific bean (or instead substitute in any phase-specific fish).

Phase 2 is the most challenging for vegetarians because it is the low-carb phase, and we aren't eating soy or soy-based products on this diet; but as long as you are willing to eat eggs and fish, you should be fine for those two Phase 2 days. Your food choices will be more limited, but it's only for two days. If you aren't willing to eat fish or eggs, see the section that follows on following the plan if you're vegan.

VEGAN

It's easy to be vegan during Phases 1 and 3 because you can always substitute legumes for meat in any recipe. However, Phase 2 is more challenging. Protein-rich legumes and grains are just too high in carbohydrates for Phase 2. That's why, as vegans, you get to break *one rule*. Just one. The soy rule.

Normally, I forbid soy on the Fast Metabolism Diet because of its plant estrogens and also because of how processed and genetically modified it tends to be. However, if you are vegan, I don't want you to feel like you can't do this diet. Therefore, during Phase 2, you may replace any meat with any of the following (but no other soy products):

- Organic, non-GMO tofu

- Organic, non-GMO soy tempeh

- Organic, non-GMO edamame

Cook the tofu without fat and grill or bake it yourself, rather than buying pre-baked tofu, which is more processed. Your weight loss might slow down somewhat, but you can still eat low-carb for those two Phase 2 days if you stick to these three options. But remember, during Phase 1 and Phase 3, you have to follow the rules just like everybody else: and that means *no soy*.

GLUTEN-FREE

Gluten-free is easy on the Fast Metabolism Diet because wheat, the main source of gluten in most people's diets, is already off the menu. However, there are a few gluten-containing products in the recipes and on the shopping lists. Don't eat them. Sprouted-grain bread and products containing spelt, barley, kamut, farro, durum, bulgur, rye, triticale, or semolina *all contain gluten*, so avoid those. Conventional oatmeal also contains gluten.

Instead, use gluten-free oatmeal (check the package—it must be processed differently to avoid contamination from wheat) and any of the gluten-free grains. These include:

- Amaranth
- Brown rice
- Buckwheat
- Millet
- Quinoa
- Teff
- Wild rice

And when using the recipes, simply substitute a gluten-free grain for whatever grain is off the meal map for you. For example, if a recipe includes barley, replace it with brown rice or quinoa. All of the gluten-free grains above are on the food list for Phase 1.

YOUR PREFERENCES

What kind of eater are you? Picky eaters may not like every recipe in this book, and they might not like every item on the grocery lists, but as long as you follow the phase-specific meal map and eat from the phase-specific list (even if you only like a few things), you'll be fine. Just be sure you eat the designated number of grains, proteins, fruits, vegetables, and fats for each meal in each phase, and never skip a meal or snack. Other than that, the food choices are up to you.

Maybe you like to eat exactly the same thing every day. No problem! Even if you have the same breakfast every day during Phase 1, that's still only eight breakfasts in a month that are the same. You're still getting plenty of variety. Or maybe you get bored easily and you like to change it up. No problem. Make something new every day, if that's what you prefer.

You don't like any of my recipes? (I don't really believe you because I think they're fantastic.) So use your own recipes, if you prefer. I promise not to be offended. As long as you adhere to the meal map and your current phase list, the diet will still work.

YOUR FAMILY

Some of my clients have families and have to cook for a spouse, partner, and/or children. One of the great things about Fast Metabolism is that it's full of real food most people like, so chances are your family will eat what you are eating. Many of the recipes in this book serve four or six, so if you have a family to feed, share your delicious meal. It's a healthy way to eat for anyone—man, woman, or child. My children love the recipes in this book and were eager taste-testers while I was perfecting them.

However, if you know your family won't like the foods you are eating, you don't have to be a short-order cook. Just do what many of my clients (and I) do: spend a day cooking for the weeks ahead. Because of the way the diet is set up, it's easy to cook four weeks' worth of meals at a time. Portion out chili, stews, rice bowls, and oatmeal into individually sized freezer containers, mark with the appropriate phase, and stack them in your freezer. Then, you can make dinner for your family and if it doesn't conform to your phase, all you have to do is defrost an appropriate meal for yourself.

YOUR COOKING STYLE

Some people love to cook and some people avoid the kitchen at all costs. The Fast Metabolism Diet is an ideal diet for foodies and people who love to cook because the recipes are interesting (but easy), flavorful, and fun to make. If you don't like to cook, dread cooking, fear any diet that requires it, then we need to talk.

One of the most important ways to get your metabolism back on track and burning fat again is to get back to real food. You remember food—that stuff in the produce aisle, behind the meat counter, and *not* partitioned and packaged up in a frozen box? Eating real food is *so important* for the repair process we have to accomplish. I really want you to take a leap of faith with me and try cooking.

The great news is that you don't have to cook very much. The recipes in this book make a lot of food, and they are specifically designed so you can make a meal and then pack up and freeze multiple additional meals (label them by phase and put them in the freezer and you're ready to go). Then, when that phase comes around again, all you have to do is take your container out of the freezer, heat it up, and voilà! Convenience food that just happens to be home-cooked and full of the intense nutrition this program requires.

TIME-SAVING TIP

One specific way to make the cooking even easier is to eat the same things in weeks one and three, and the same things in weeks two and four. This adds plenty of variety to your meals, but keeps the cooking to a minimum. Plan for a day when you can cook all the meals for week one, then freeze the leftovers and use those meals during week three. Spend another day cooking all the meals for week two, then freeze the leftovers and have those meals during week four. It's a really efficient way to make sure you always have something good to eat. (And when you get to week three, you'll find out exactly why this is such a good idea. A little hint—you will be looking good and might want to deviate from the plan. Having already prepared foods will keep you motivated to stay on track.)

Foodie or not, cooking savvy or not, cooking ahead like this will save you a lot of time and aggravation. In fact, I rely heavily on my freezer, as well as my three slow cookers and my stockpot. Sometimes I'll have four different recipes going at the same time. It's a nice way to spend a Sunday, if you like to cook the way I do. But even if you don't, let me assure you again that these recipes are easy. No fancy techniques. They mostly involve chopping some things and putting everything together in a pot or slow cooker, then letting it cook until it's done. Plus, you can console yourself, knowing you won't have to cook anything else for weeks.

Week One requires the most cooking, but again, you'll make enough to carry you through future weeks. Some of my clients like to cook for the whole 28 days at once, and this is not so hard to do. Or, just cook when you have time, and pack up the leftovers. Then, all you have to do is deal out your meals like a deck of cards (unless family members pilfer your frozen meals because they taste so good—that happens to me all the time).

Worth noting is that, of course, you don't have to cook ahead. If you love to cook and you have time to prepare all your meals from scratch before you eat them, then go for it! But time can be a problem, even for those of us who like to cook. Cooking ahead helps with the time factor, too. But again, work to your preferences and needs; if you don't want to, you don't have to cook a bunch of meals at once. Maybe you have time to make dinner one evening, so you make chicken stew. Make extra, enjoy it, and freeze the rest. Always keep thinking about how you can make future meals easier. Do it the way it works in your life. But please don't fear cooking. It's crucial to your health and the metabolic changes we're instigating. You can do this!

Cooking is a small price to pay for restored health and the body of your dreams. Home-cooked food is the most nutritious, so it feeds your body with what it needs to work better. It also has the pleasant side effect of making you, and your family, feel nurtured and healthy. So get cooking, crocking, simmering, baking, no matter what your style!

BUDGET FRIENDLY

Cooking ahead and freezing meals is budget-friendly, but there are other ways to make Fast Metabolism cost-effective. Instead of varying every meal or snack, which would require you to buy a lot of different foods and use just a few of them, some of my clients prefer to stick to one or two snacks and meals throughout the course of the 28 days. Buy in bulk and package up nuts, seeds, or spelt pretzels. Make a big batch of chili and have it for several meals each week. If you don't mind sticking to a few trusty meals and snacks, you'll save a lot of money and you won't have a lot of wasted food.

YOUR ACTIVITY LEVEL

Finally, let's talk about exercise. The Fast Metabolism Diet is designed to include three days of exercise per week:

- One day of cardio in Phase 1

- One day of strength-training in Phase 2

- One day of yoga, stretching, or deep-breathing in Phase 3

That means you can do the treadmill or spin class during Phase 1, a Body Pump class during Phase 2, and your Vinyasa or Bikram yoga class during Phase 3. If you don't belong to a gym, you can take a brisk walk or run around the neighborhood during Phase 1. During Phase 2, you can lift weights at home, even if you just have a set of dumbbells. During Phase 3, do a yoga or stretching DVD, or check out some of the great deep-breathing exercises on YouTube. Just remember: Don't mix and match your exercises. They are phase-specific, too, like your food lists.

If you haven't been exercising at all, the three days is all you have to do.

What if you are an exercise fanatic? I've had clients tell me, "But I go to spin class *every day!*" or "I do Boot Camp class five days a week!"

This is what I say: "Not for the next 28 days you don't."

We're programmed to believe that the more we exercise, the faster we'll lose weight, but the very nature of exercise is to break and tear down the muscles, and then to use the body's resources to repair them. I'm being greedy with your resources right now. I want you to channel all that energy into repairing the metabolism, not torn-down muscles. Three days of exercise per week is all you need to help boost your metabolism, while also conserving the energy from the foods you are eating to use it for metabolism repair.

If you are someone who exercises every day, and you just don't feel right if you aren't doing it, then you can work it into the plan. You have to match the exercise to the phase, though, still. You can do cardio, but only during Phase 1. That means two days of cardio per week, including spin class, aerobics class, dance classes like Jazzercise or Zumba, running, or jogging or cardio machines at the gym, like the elliptical trainer or treadmill. It's only for 28 days, and two cardio days per week when you are eating the most carb-rich and sugar-rich foods is enough to maintain your fitness level.

You can do weight lifting for two days per week, too, but only during Phase 2. Do upper-body lifting on one of the days, and lower-body lifting on the other day, if you want to lift on both days.

During Phase 3, you can do yoga on all three days, if you like. As I said earlier, for the plan to be effective, once is enough. But if you have to have more exercise, it's yoga or stretching classes only. Also, be sure to end with a nice, long relaxation period that includes deep breathing, to calm your body. When the 28 days are over, you can go back to your normal exercise routine. Remember, exercise stresses the body. So pay attention to how you feel while exercising and take care of yourself. Do enough to help, but not so much that you hurt.

PERSONALIZING AND BUILDING YOUR OWN MEAL MAPS

Some clients want a meal map to follow, period. That's why I provide you with an ideal meal map of suggested foods in the next four chapters, for each of the upcoming four weeks of the Fast Metabolism Diet. For many clients, however, a more personalized approach sometimes works better, so I've provided this section for those who'd like to fill out their own maps for the next four weeks.

The meal map will be your guide for keeping track of your day, like when you get up, what phase it is, and what you will be eating. Your personalized meal map will allow you to fill in the foods *you* love to eat, while still staying within each phase. Use the phase-specific food lists from the last chapter or refer to the Master Food Lists at the back of the book to decide what you want ahead of time. Then, when your week begins, you'll have everything you'll need, and you'll know exactly what to eat—and you can be assured it will be foods you already know you like.

When I meet with clients, I help them do this. We spend a lot of time filling out their meal maps based on their preferences. I like to ask them:

What foods do you love? I have them highlight all the foods they already know they love on the food list for that phase, and then circle the foods they would like to try. Then I have them look over the food lists and cross off anything they don't like.

Next, we fill out the meal map. I like to start in pencil and always begin with snacks. Working from the phase-appropriate lists, we fill in the snacks you know you will like. Then we go to the breakfasts and dinners. Finally, we do the lunches because these are good for leftovers from either breakfast or dinner—like crumbling leftover turkey bacon from breakfast on your salad for lunch, or having a filet for dinner and saving just enough for a steak lettuce wrap for the next day.

MUST-DO: STRATEGIC SNACKS!

Snacks are the things people tend to leave out or forget most often, but they are absolutely vital for success on this program. Snacks are the kindling for the metabolic fire, so the body can better digest and metabolize the meals. Each snack is strategically placed and each snack type is strategically chosen to invoke a specific neurochemical, biochemical, physiological, and metabolic response. They cannot be left out, and they must be phase-specific!

Here's a blank meal map for you to work with in creating your own personalized way of following Fast Metabolism. When you begin each week, you are going to:

1. Fill in the snacks *you like* for the entire week.

2. Fill in the breakfasts *you like* for the entire week.

3. Fill in the dinners *you like* for the entire week.

4. Fill in the lunches *you like,* using as many leftovers as you can that are in your designated phase.

WEEK-AT-A-GLANCE MEAL MAP

	WAKE TIME	WEIGHT	BREAKFAST	SNACK	LUNCH	SNACK	DINNER	EXERCISE	WATER
PHASE 1 MONDAY	__:__ am/pm	_____	__:__ am/pm	__:__ am/pm	__:__ am/pm	__:__ am/pm	__:__ am/pm		
TUESDAY	__:__ am/pm	_____	__:__ am/pm	__:__ am/pm	__:__ am/pm	__:__ am/pm	__:__ am/pm		
PHASE 2 WEDNESDAY	__:__ am/pm	_____	__:__ am/pm	__:__ am/pm	__:__ am/pm	__:__ am/pm	__:__ am/pm		
THURSDAY	__:__ am/pm	_____	__:__ am/pm	__:__ am/pm	__:__ am/pm	__:__ am/pm	__:__ am/pm		
PHASE 3 FRIDAY	__:__ am/pm	_____	__:__ am/pm	__:__ am/pm	__:__ am/pm	__:__ am/pm	__:__ am/pm		
SATURDAY	__:__ am/pm	_____	__:__ am/pm	__:__ am/pm	__:__ am/pm	__:__ am/pm	__:__ am/pm		
SUNDAY	__:__ am/pm	_____	__:__ am/pm	__:__ am/pm	__:__ am/pm	__:__ am/pm	__:__ am/pm		

BLANK MEAL MAP, *PHASE 1*

PHASE 1: UNWIND STRESS

WAKE TIME	WEIGHT	BREAKFAST	SNACK	LUNCH	SNACK	DINNER	EXERCISE	WATER
_:_ am/pm **MONDAY**	___	_:_ am/pm P1 GRAIN P1 FRUIT	_:_ am/pm P1 FRUIT	_:_ am/pm P1 GRAIN P1 PROTEIN P1 FRUIT P1 VEGGIE	_:_ am/pm P1 FRUIT	_:_ am/pm P1 GRAIN P1 VEGGIE P1 PROTEIN		
_:_ am/pm **TUESDAY**	___	_:_ am/pm P1 GRAIN P1 FRUIT	_:_ am/pm P1 FRUIT	_:_ am/pm P1 GRAIN P1 PROTEIN P1 FRUIT P1 VEGGIE	_:_ am/pm P1 FRUIT	_:_ am/pm P1 GRAIN P1 VEGGIE P1 PROTEIN		

BLANK MEAL MAP, *PHASE 2*

	PHASE 2: UNLOCK FAT							
WAKE TIME	WEIGHT	BREAKFAST	SNACK	LUNCH	SNACK	DINNER	EXERCISE	WATER
__:__ am/pm **WEDNESDAY**	_____	__:__ am/pm **P2 PROTEIN** **P2 VEGGIE**	__:__ am/pm **P2 PROTEIN**	__:__ am/pm **P2 PROTEIN** **P2 VEGGIE**	__:__ am/pm **P2 PROTEIN**	__:__ am/pm **P2 PROTEIN** **P2 VEGGIE**		
__:__ am/pm **THURSDAY**	_____	__:__ am/pm **P2 PROTEIN** **P2 VEGGIE**	__:__ am/pm **P2 PROTEIN**	__:__ am/pm **P2 PROTEIN** **P2 VEGGIE**	__:__ am/pm **P2 PROTEIN**	__:__ am/pm **P2 PROTEIN** **P2 VEGGIE**		

BLANK MEAL MAP, PHASE 3

PHASE 3: UNLEASH YOUR METABOLISM

	WAKE TIME	WEIGHT	BREAKFAST	SNACK	LUNCH	SNACK	DINNER	EXERCISE	WATER
FRIDAY	__:__ am/pm	___	__:__ am/pm P3 FRUIT P3 HEALTHY FAT/PROTEIN P3 GRAIN P3 VEGGIE	__:__ am/pm P3 HEALTHY FAT/PROTEIN P3 VEGGIE	__:__ am/pm P3 HEALTHY FAT/PROTEIN P3 VEGGIE P3 FRUIT	__:__ am/pm P3 HEALTHY FAT/PROTEIN P3 VEGGIE (OPTIONAL)	__:__ am/pm P3 HEALTHY FAT/PROTEIN P3 VEGGIE P3 GRAIN (OPTIONAL)		
SATURDAY	__:__ am/pm	___	__:__ am/pm P3 FRUIT P3 HEALTHY FAT/PROTEIN P3 GRAIN P3 VEGGIE	__:__ am/pm P3 HEALTHY FAT/PROTEIN P3 VEGGIE	__:__ am/pm P3 HEALTHY FAT/PROTEIN P3 VEGGIE P3 FRUIT	__:__ am/pm P3 HEALTHY FAT/PROTEIN P3 VEGGIE (OPTIONAL)	__:__ am/pm P3 VEGGIE P3 HEALTHY FAT/PROTEIN P3 GRAIN (OPTIONAL)		
SUNDAY	__:__ am/pm	___	__:__ am/pm P3 FRUIT P3 HEALTHY FAT/PROTEIN P3 GRAIN P3 VEGGIE	__:__ am/pm P3 HEALTHY FAT/PROTEIN P3 VEGGIE	__:__ am/pm P3 HEALTHY FAT/PROTEIN P3 VEGGIE P3 FRUIT	__:__ am/pm P3 HEALTHY FAT/PROTEIN P3 VEGGIE (OPTIONAL)	__:__ am/pm P3 HEALTHY FAT/PROTEIN P3 VEGGIE P3 GRAIN (OPTIONAL)		

All done. Wasn't that kind of fun? By doing this, you will create your own diet totally based on how you live and what you like to eat.

The keys to success on the Fast Metabolism Diet are to know the rules, know yourself, and plan ahead. Make time for pre-cooking, stock up on freezer containers, and commit. Craft the diet around who you are and what you do, and then get ready to feel better than you've felt for a long time.

BEFORE YOU TURN THE PAGE

The next four chapters are set up to walk you through some of the emotional landmines and pitfalls that may pop up along the way during the next four weeks, as well as to take you through proven "ideal" meal maps for those who don't want to craft their own. I've discovered, after years of taking clients through this plan, that each week has some unique characteristics in terms of what you are likely to experience and feel. Let's look at the landscape and see what you can do to keep feeding your body and your brain to keep your metabolism ignited throughout this process.

Part III:
Four Weeks
to Fabulous

CHAPTER SIX

HAYLIE
POMROY

Week One: Freefall

Welcome to week one! This week, we're going to take your body through all three phases of the Fast Metabolism Diet. You'll be on Phase 1 for two days, Phase 2 for two days, and Phase 3 for three days. You're going to eat a lot of food, and some of it may seem too good to be true. You might not love everything, but you're learning this week what you do and don't like in each phase. You're going to learn a lot.

I know you're excited to get started, and I'm ready to talk you through it, every step of the way. In this chapter, you're going to fill out your first official meal map, and you're going to fill it out with all the meals and snacks you get to eat this week. Or, if you just want me to tell you what to eat, you can go by the Week One Ideal Meal Map that I've already prepared for you. I find that some of my clients want me to tell them exactly what to eat, while others want to figure it all out for themselves. Whichever one describes you, you've got the tools.

So let's talk about week one, what I like to call Freefall Week.

FREEFALL WEEK—WHAT TO EXPECT, WHAT YOU'RE LIKELY TO FEEL

Week one is exciting, but because this is so different, it can also be confusing and a little scary. Remember, I want to confuse your metabolism, but

I don't want to confuse *you*. But in beginning the plan, you're about to go through a lot of changes. This new way of eating might take a little getting used to at first.

Also, you may have to make peace with your old food demons. As you prepare to begin the diet, they may rear their ugly heads. Your former obsessions with calorie counting or carb counting, your fear of fruit or meat or fat, your past failures—all of it is likely to come to the table. Hear my words: they are unwelcome guests for this feast. Freefall with me and check those old demons at the door. I want you to be ready for this, I want you to understand what's happening and I want you to know you are not alone on this journey.

Here are some of the things I hear from my clients right before they begin week one:

- I can't lose weight with that many carbs.

- I lost weight before on Diet XYZ, and this doesn't sound anything like Diet XYZ.

- I can't stick to diets. I have no willpower.

- I'm afraid I won't like the food!

- What if I eat too much for it to work?

- What if I don't lose weight the first week?

What if? What if? What if???!

I get a lot of skeptics at the beginning, so the biggest thing I tell people for week one is to *trust*. Let go of your preconceived ideas and past diet history. Let go of being so vested in how you think your body will or won't react to this diet. You don't *know* what will happen. You haven't even started. I'm asking you to freefall a little bit this week, to let yourself go and dive into this. Recognize how much you are asking of your body. Notice the paradigm shift, but don't get worked up about it or let it freak you out. Let the plan feel easy. Yes, it's a little scary, but I need you to just let go, trust it and commit to doing it, even if you don't know exactly what to expect. Even though you're nervous, or a little bit scared.

I'm a firm believer in positive affirmations. This week, even before you begin, visualize yourself losing weight, setting goals, but not getting too vested in the numbers. Really focus on the repair that's happening and the changes you can detect in your body. We're going to be asking a lot of your body this week, metabolically. We're asking the body to jump up and pay attention. It's not only a mental and emotional paradigm shift, but a huge metabolic paradigm shift, so your past success or failure will have nothing to do with what you are doing now. This is a whole new ball game.

A LOT OF A LOT

Another thing I warn my clients about for week one is that this week, you're going to have to get used to having a lot of a lot. What I mean is that on some days, you're going to have a lot of fruit. On other days, you're going to have a lot of protein. On some days, you'll have a lot of vegetables. On other days, you'll have a lot of fat. "A lot" is designed to enrich the body, giving it the nutrients it needs so that it can manufacture things like muscle, bone, hair, skin, and nails. Don't forget our main goal here: to transform the metabolism so we can actually extract the nutrients from our food and use them to create health and hormone stabilization.

That being said, you are likely to see a good chunk of weight loss this week. Most of my clients lose anywhere from half a pound to a pound a day, and sometimes a little more. That can feel scary, too. Some people wonder if it's happening too fast, if they are burning muscle instead of fat. Others are impatient and think it isn't happening fast enough, or they fear they aren't being successful enough.

It's okay, even a good thing, to be a little bit passive this week. Don't read too much into what happens. Don't get all worked up about the numbers right now. Instead, focus your energy and mindset on nailing the rhythm of the phases and getting into and comfortable with your grocery list. Really pay attention to the differences in the foods you are eating during each phase. Take note of the foods you enjoy most, and highlight them on your grocery list. Take notes. Participate in the repair of your own health. You're just getting a handle on the flow, so be mentally engaged, but not anxious. If you follow the rules I've laid out and trust the diet, the rest will work itself out.

Once we get into the week, I hear a lot more positives coming from my clients, especially about the food. Things like:

"Oh, that's right, I forgot how much I love mangos!"

"Don't ever take my rice crackers away, I can't believe I can have those."

"I love this filet mignon phase!"

"That coconut curry was my favorite."

If you don't like something, don't worry about it. You don't have to eat it again. Don't get hung up on what you don't like. So you bought almond butter and you don't like it, and now you're fretting about how you paid for a whole jar of almond butter that you aren't going to eat. You've got to let that stuff go. You're learning. And plenty of people like almond butter, so give it to a friend who does. Everything's going to be just fine. And remember, stress hormones increase fat storage. So let it go. . . .

Focus on the things that really stand out to you as delicious—how good the fruit is and how great you feel after eating it compared to your old starchy or refined sugary snacks. Focus on the luxury of a nice cut of meat, or of getting to slather everything on your plate with avocado. Remember those five major players need you and need these foods to repair and heal. You can do this! And I am so proud of you for feeding your metabolism.

This is just the beginning. It's going to be life changing.

DON'T FORGET TO DO PHASE-APPROPRIATE EXERCISE:

At least one day of gentle to moderate cardio during Phase 1

At least one day of heavy weight lifting during Phase 2

At least one day of ultra-relaxing activity in Phase 3, like yoga, a walk outdoors on a nice day, or a massage. In fact, I strongly recommend scheduling a massage in particular for Phase 3 of week one, to help soothe your body into the new routine.

WHAT TO EAT THIS WEEK:
YOUR DAILY MEAL MAP FOR WEEK ONE

When my clients come into my office we create meal maps for the week so they know exactly what to eat at any given moment. This planning ahead makes the program a no-brainer and so easy to follow. I've created a meal map below for you. All the meals have already been filled out. You can switch meals within phases, or use some of these meals but not others. As long as you are sticking to the phase-specific foods and categories for each meal and snack, and your portions are correct, you can always adapt this to your own needs. (See "Personalizing and Building Your Own Meal Maps," page 116, for step-by-step instructions on crafting your own meal map.)

Notice that each phase is highlighted. I've written the meal components above, and in a line below, the foods or recipes that can work for that meal. Foods with recipes in the back of the book are written in bold and have been labeled according to their phase.

Remember, this will involve some cooking, but don't be afraid! Whenever you make a recipe, pack up additional servings, label them with the appropriate phase, and put them in the freezer. I've designed these meal maps so that many of the recipes from this first week pop up again in the "ideal" meal map I give you for week three. So when they do, you'll already have all the cooking finished! Take advantage of your excitement and momentum this week to get all your cooking done now, in case the novelty wears off in another week or two.

Also a reminder: This is a meal map for someone whose weight loss goal is 20 pounds or less. For every additional 20 pounds you need to lose, increase your portions by one-half serving. (For example, if you need to lose 20 pounds, a serving of chili is 2 cups. If you need to lose 40 pounds, a serving of chili is 3 cups.)

WEEK ONE MEAL MAP, *PHASE 1*

PHASE 1: UNWIND STRESS

WAKE TIME	WEIGHT	BREAKFAST	SNACK	LUNCH	SNACK	DINNER	EXERCISE	WATER
__:__ am/pm **MONDAY**	___	__:__ am/pm P1 OATMEAL FRUIT SMOOTHIE	__:__ am/pm 1 ASIAN PEAR	__:__ am/pm P1 OPEN-FACED TURKEY SANDWICH, 1 ORANGE	__:__ am/pm 2 KIWIS	__:__ am/pm P1 CHICKEN AND BARLEY SOUP		
__:__ am/pm **TUESDAY**	___	__:__ am/pm STRAWBERRY FRENCH TOAST	__:__ am/pm 1 APPLE	__:__ am/pm P1 CHICKEN AND BARLEY SOUP, SLICED KIWI	__:__ am/pm 1 CUP WATERMELON CUBES	__:__ am/pm P1 CHILI		

WEEK ONE MEAL MAP, PHASE 2

PHASE 2: UNLOCK FAT

WAKE TIME	WEIGHT	BREAKFAST	SNACK	LUNCH	SNACK	DINNER	EXERCISE	WATER
__:__ am/pm **WEDNESDAY**	___	__:__ am/pm P2 SPANISH EGG WHITE SCRAMBLE	__:__ am/pm SMOKED SALMON WITH CUCUMBERS	__:__ am/pm P2 TUNA AND CUCUMBER SALAD	__:__ am/pm 1 TO 2 OUNCES BUFFALO JERKY	__:__ am/pm P2 STEAK AND ASPARAGUS LETTUCE WRAP		
__:__ am/pm **THURSDAY**	___	__:__ am/pm P2 TURKEY BACON WITH CELERY	__:__ am/pm P2 STUFFED MUSHROOMS	__:__ am/pm P2 STEAK AND SPINACH SALAD	__:__ am/pm 3 HARD-BOILED EGG WHITES WITH SEA SALT AND PEPPER	__:__ am/pm P2 PEPPERONCINI PORK ROAST, 2 CUPS BROCCOLI		

WEEK ONE MEAL MAP, *PHASE 3*

	WAKE TIME	WEIGHT	BREAKFAST	SNACK	LUNCH	SNACK	DINNER	EXERCISE	WATER
FRIDAY	__:__ am/pm	____	__:__ am/pm P3 BERRY NUTTY OATMEAL	__:__ am/pm ⅓ CUP HUMMUS AND CUCUMBERS	__:__ am/pm P3 THREE-EGG SALAD OVER 2 CUPS SPINACH, BLUEBERRIES	__:__ am/pm ¼ CUP RAW ALMONDS	__:__ am/pm P3 SHRIMP AND VEGGIE STIR-FRY OVER ½ CUP QUINOA		
SATURDAY	__:__ am/pm	____	__:__ am/pm P3 TOAST, BERRIES, NUT BUTTER, CUCUMBERS	__:__ am/pm ¼ CUP RAW PISTACHIOS	__:__ am/pm P3 SHRIMP AND VEGGIE STIR-FRY, WITHOUT THE PASTA, ½ GRAPEFRUIT	__:__ am/pm ½ SLICED AVOCADO WITH SEA SALT	__:__ am/pm AVOCADO AND TURKEY LETTUCE WRAP		
SUNDAY	__:__ am/pm	____	__:__ am/pm P3 TOAST, EGG, TOMATO, RED ONION, ½ AVOCADO	__:__ am/pm ⅓ CUP HUMMUS AND CUCUMBERS	__:__ am/pm P3 ENDIVE TUNA SALAD, APPLE	__:__ am/pm CELERY AND 2 TABLESPOONS RAW ALMOND BUTTER	__:__ am/pm P3 COCONUT CURRY CHICKEN		

Remember, this is *our* plan. My rules, your preferences. You can be as creative as you like, within the guidelines. Follow one of my plans, or a plan entirely your own. You are taking your health into your own hands, so get ready, get set, and go! Think of it as a puzzle, a challenge, and most of all, this week, just trust it. Freefall. The Fast Metabolism Diet will catch you.

HAYLIE
POMROY

Week Two: OMG!

You've done a whole week on the Fast Metabolism Diet. You've gone through all three phases once, and I know you are feeling different from how you did a week ago. Now, welcome to week two!

This week, we're going to take your body through all three phases of the Fast Metabolism Diet again, but it won't be the same as last week because you are in a different week of your own, individual four-week cycle (girls and guys). You're exposing a *different* body to the three phases this week, and this is where it starts to get exciting! This week you bring to the table a body that has soothed its adrenals and stimulated its liver. A body that has nurtured the production of thyroid and other fat-burning hormones and a body that is beginning to change its composition, converting fat to fuel and fuel to muscle. And just imagine the pituitary being all atwitter as it orchestrates all of these glorious events!

By now, you've lost some weight, so you might be starting to see the light. Your inner skeptic may be quieting down. In this chapter, I'm going to talk you through the week again and you'll get a brand-new meal map (whether you follow the one I provide here or fill out your own, that's entirely up to you).

I also want to talk to you about what's going to happen during this week. Last week was the freefall chapter. You had to take a leap of faith and trust in the diet. Now, it's getting real. I often call this the "Oh Sh*t Week," but some folks might not like that, so I've edited myself a bit (just a bit) . . .

OMG! WEEK—WHAT TO EXPECT, WHAT YOU'RE LIKELY TO FEEL

Week two is always an interesting one. Often, people start to freak out a little about what just happened and what is going to happen next. Week two can be a bit of a roller-coaster ride, both emotionally and organizationally. OMG, you haven't been on the program long enough for it to feel like second nature and haven't quite gotten the rhythm of it all down pat, but all you know is that it's *exciting*! Also, you might be excited or afraid or even confused about how your body is reacting to the program. Have you lost enough weight? Lost too much weight? Finally coming out of your coffee and refined sugar withdrawals only to find you don't even remember much of last week? Let's take a collective deep breath and soldier on, letting the program tether us to continuity, consistency, and repair. The momentum will increase this next week, so don't fight it or get too creative—just stick with the flow. People usually react to this scary feeling of increasing momentum in one of two ways: terrified the weight loss is going to stop if they restrict their portions or they double up on their servings thinking they can go rogue and experience the same weight loss.

A lot of my clients see significant weight loss in week one, and sometimes they are terrified that it's going to stop. They think maybe it was just a fluke or sheer luck or not sustainable. They often react by cutting their portions. They pull back their protein servings to 3 ounces and their vegetable servings to ½ cup at dinner, eating nothing but protein and veggies in Phase 1, leaving out the critical grain. Or they skip their fruit at breakfast in Phase 3, thinking that less food will give them even more weight loss. This is exactly the wrong thing to do if you are trying to heat up your metabolism.

The other way they react is to say something like this to themselves, "Oh, my gosh, I've lost so much weight, this can't be healthy, I better eat more." Or, "Hey, if I can lose that much weight doing exactly what Haylie says, then I should be able to eat even more and it is okay if I don't lose as much in the second week!" Then they go rogue and start cheating, adding carbs or fats in the wrong places and phases, until they slide back into their old habits.

Both of these dysfunctional strategies will stop weight loss in its tracks.

I had a client who had significant weight loss in her first week. She had been an angel and it had paid off big time. During week two, her food diary showed that she had pulled a lot of the grain servings out of her meal map in Phase 1, and left the avocado off her toast in Phase 3. She even skipped a 3:00 snack because she wasn't hungry. She thought, "If I'm doing this well and I'm this full and this satisfied, just imagine what I could do if I took more food away!" She then decided to do four spin classes and an intense run in a span of five days. When we sat down together at the end of week two, she had only lost a pound and was feeling pretty ragged out. I couldn't believe how easy it was for me to convince her to begin the whole program over—that's right, we started from scratch! She went on to have a glorious, satisfied, successful four weeks and saw a lot more of her massage therapist and a lot less of her spin instructor.

Because my client had limited so much of the food and had increased her intense exercise, I was concerned that her starvation-mode hormones would be in full swing. If the body goes into starvation mode, that will increase stress hormones. And what do stress hormones do? They signal the body to store fat rather than burn it. So this week, be so gentle with yourself and be mindful of stress.

Stress is definitely a factor in week two—this is exactly why I call it the OMG week! People get stressed about how much weight they lost, about whether their weight loss is fast enough or too fast. Or, they go in the opposite direction, wondering whether their excessive weight loss means they can start changing the rules of the plan.

It's important to understand that while guilt is fattening and stress is fattening, feeling guilty about being stressed is the most fattening of all! So get massages this week, take a hot bath in lavender oil, try to take your cardio outside at the beach or a park, and be prepared with your food because it is what will coast you through. I once had a client who, with great anxiety, told me that he was almost all the way through a pear he had grabbed as a quick snack when he realized he was in Phase 2. "I panicked!" he said. Don't panic; just be prepared.

During week two, make a conscious effort to let stress and guilt *go*. Stress evokes hormone responses we don't want right now, so if you have slipped or mixed up phases, don't stress. Just move forward with greater consciousness. The best thing you can do for yourself, besides sticking to the plan, is to keep feeling great about what you are doing. Feel empowered, feel strong, and if you make a mistake, forgive yourself and move on. Feeling guilty only compounds any slipup.

These common feelings are usually based in fear about what just happened the week before and disbelief that you can actually enjoy eating and still lose weight, or thinking last week was a fluke and there is no way that it can happen two weeks in a row. Sometimes, I even see this type of thinking begin to happen at the tail end of week one.

Listen to these very important words: *True metabolism repair happens when we have stability and consistency in our repair process.*

Every phase in this plan is intense and focused, which is why it requires a lot of energy from the body, and why we can only stay on it for a short period of time. If we do a phase for too long, the body gets exhausted and can't do the necessary work. This is why we change the phases in the way we do. But you can't mess with them or start improvising, or the process is going to stop working.

Week two is your chance to nail down the rhythm that you established in week one. It is definitely not the time to start changing anything. Stability and consistency reduce stress in all aspects of your life, physiologically and mentally, so your body feels that it's okay to burn fat because it's no longer necessary to hoard it. Just stick with the program. It's all going to work out great.

So, during week two, you may be thinking, "OMG, I have to change something to keep this going," or "OMG, I have to change something to slow down this run-away weight-loss train," but stop. Take a deep, calming breath. Week two is about *not* making any drastic changes.

Instead, what I would like you to focus on in week two is celebrating what you enjoyed from the previous week, and maybe being open to trying new and different foods you didn't try last week. It's also a good week to get a little bit curious about what is happening in your body. Approach it with wonder rather than fear. If the first week was about trusting, this week is more about being inquisitive and staying open.

Try not to have a knee-jerk reaction to what happened in the first week. Approach it with an open mind. Your body is responding to some pretty amazing metabolic changes, so in week two, you have to convince your body that: *Yes, we're really going to do this and yes, we really have everything we need. We have enough fruit, enough fat, enough carbs, enough protein. I'm not going to choke you by putting in too much and I'm not going to starve you by taking too much away. We will have enough.* This is what your body needs to feel, and the best way to transmit this message from your brain to your metabolism is by calming down, paying attention, and toeing the line.

EACH WORKOUT HAS A PURPOSE

Don't forget your phase-appropriate exercise! One day of gentle to moderate cardio during Phase 1, but this week try to take it outside or do a dance class with music you love. Have at least one day of heavy weight lifting during Phase 2 and really pump some iron, maybe even with loud rock music on your headphones, leaving any stress or frustration the week has offered you in a pool of sweat at the gym. And also remember to do at least one day of ultra-relaxing activity in Phase 3, like a mellow yoga class, or go get that massage. I have found that many of the massage schools give free or deeply discounted massages, and they are typically very good because the students are trying to impress an instructor. If you're feeling good and you want to do more, that's fine. Just keep it phase-specific. You can do two cardio days during Phase 1, but don't do cardio during Phases 2 or 3. Stick to weight lifting in Phase 2 and stress-reducing activities in Phase 3. Exercise increases endorphins, the feel-good hormones, and as you cross-train your meal map again this week you will be stimulating, rebuilding, and replenishing each of your five major players, as well as bringing balance to that brain-flesh-hormone connection.

Here's an example of an ideal meal map for week two. As always, you can substitute, as long as you stick to your phase.

WEEK TWO MEAL MAP, *PHASE 1*

PHASE 1: UNWIND STRESS

	WAKE TIME	WEIGHT	BREAKFAST	SNACK	LUNCH	SNACK	DINNER	EXERCISE	WATER
MONDAY	__:__ am/pm	_____	__:__ am/pm P1 STRAWBERRY FRENCH TOAST	__:__ am/pm 2 APRICOTS	__:__ am/pm P1 TUNA, GREEN APPLE, AND SPINACH SALAD 1 SLICE SPROUTED GRAIN BREAD	__:__ am/pm 1 CUP CANTALOUPE	__:__ am/pm P1 CHICKEN SAUSAGE WITH BROWN RICE FUSILLI		
TUESDAY	__:__ am/pm	_____	__:__ am/pm P1 OATMEAL FRUIT SMOOTHIE	__:__ am/pm 1 CUP MANGO SLICES	__:__ am/pm P1 CHICKEN SAUSAGE WITH BROWN RICE FUSILLI, 1 ASIAN PEAR	__:__ am/pm 1 ORANGE	__:__ am/pm P1 PORK TENDERLOIN WITH BROCCOLI		

WEEK TWO MEAL MAP, PHASE 2

PHASE 2: UNLOCK FAT

WAKE TIME	WEIGHT	BREAKFAST	SNACK	LUNCH	SNACK	DINNER	EXERCISE	WATER
WEDNESDAY ___:___ am/pm	_____	___:___ am/pm P2 SPANISH EGG WHITE SCRAMBLE	___:___ am/pm P2 ROAST BEEF, HORSERADISH, AND CUCUMBER WRAP	___:___ am/pm P2 TUNA SALAD–STUFFED RED PEPPER	___:___ am/pm 2 OUNCES TURKEY JERKY	___:___ am/pm P2 NEW YORK STRIP STEAK WITH STEAMED BROCCOLI		
THURSDAY ___:___ am/pm	_____	___:___ am/pm P2 EGG WHITE, MUSHROOM, AND SPINACH OMELET	___:___ am/pm P2 SMOKED SALMON AND CUCUMBERS	___:___ am/pm P2 STEAK AND SPINACH SALAD (USE LEFTOVER STEAK FROM LAST NIGHT'S DINNER)	___:___ am/pm 3 HARD-BOILED EGG WHITES WITH SEA SALT AND PEPPER	___:___ am/pm P2 BEEF AND CABBAGE SOUP		

WEEK TWO MEAL MAP, PHASE 3

PHASE 3: UNLEASH YOUR METABOLISM

WAKE TIME	WEIGHT	BREAKFAST	SNACK	LUNCH	SNACK	DINNER	EXERCISE	WATER
FRIDAY ___:___ am/pm	___	___:___ am/pm P3 CUCUMBER HUMMUS TOAST, ½ GRAPEFRUIT	___:___ am/pm ¼ CUP RAW NUTS WITH LIME, SEA SALT, AND JICAMA	___:___ am/pm P3 ENDIVE TUNA SALAD 1 PEACH	___:___ am/pm ¼ CUP RAW PISTACHIOS	___:___ am/pm P3 ROSEMARY PORK ROAST WITH SWEET POTATO		
SATURDAY ___:___ am/pm	___	___:___ am/pm BERRY NUTTY OATMEAL SMOOTHIE P3 VEGGIE	___:___ am/pm ¼ CUP RAW ALMONDS	___:___ am/pm P3 OLIVE AND TOMATO SALAD 1 CUP BLUEBERRIES	___:___ am/pm ½ SLICED AVOCADO WITH SEA SALT	___:___ am/pm P3 BAKED SALMON AND SWEET POTATOES		
SUNDAY ___:___ am/pm	___	___:___ am/pm P3 EGG AND TOAST WITH TOMATOES AND RED ONION	___:___ am/pm CELERY AND 2 TABLESPOONS RAW ALMOND BUTTER	___:___ am/pm P3 SHRIMP SALAD 1 CUP RASPBERRIES	___:___ am/pm P3 SWEET POTATO HUMMUS AND CUCUMBERS	___:___ am/pm P3 COCONUT PECAN-CRUSTED HALIBUT WITH ARTICHOKE DIP		

Remember, you can be as creative as you like, within the guidelines. Stay strong with the cooking because if you froze enough foods during week one, you'll hardly have to cook at all next week, unless you want to. Before you go shopping for next week's meals map, do a freezer inventory. Base your meals on what you've already got frozen—some dinners you loved? Raw almonds or frozen mangos? Figure out what you need to use up, and include it in your meal map for next week.

The weight is peeling off, and you are looking and feeling fantastic. You can probably feel that inner burn, which is fat melting away as the flame of your metabolism is stoked. Burn, baby, burn, all the way through week two!

CHAPTER EIGHT

Week Three: "If You Think I Look Good Now . . ."

After two weeks on the Fast Metabolism Diet, your weight loss is beginning to look pretty obvious to the outside world. During week three, my clients tell me that they are finally starting to get to that place where they understand what I've been telling them all along—they get it. The fear is gone and they finally believe that they really can lose weight by eating food. By now, you are comfortable with the diet. You know what you're doing. You start to hit your stride and notice that your body is responding. This is truly a transformational week, where the paradigm has actually shifted. You're believing in yourself. You're believing in your ability to heal your metabolism—and to gain a fast metabolism.

This is also the week that my clients say they start to get a lot of comments. Week three is the head-turning week. You've got a new energy and confidence, and you're looking hot. During week three, a lot of my clients also tell me that they've finally recognized how painless losing weight on the Fast Metabolism Diet really is. They can still socialize, they can still eat with other people, and they don't have to feel isolated. There are so many great food options that doing the Fast Metabolism Diet in the real world is easier than they ever imagined it would be.

However . . . this week has its own very particular challenge. I've seen it hundreds of times. I like to call this the "cocky week," or the "If You Think I Look Good Now, Wait Until You See Me With a Drink in My Hand" week.

You're down 10, maybe 14 pounds, and you're thinking, *Hey, this isn't so hard. This is my ace in the hole. If I screw off now, if I cheat a little, I can always go back to it and lose more.* So you start to cheat. You think, *Why not have a couple of glasses of wine at this party?* or *I'll just have a piece of cake, it's no big deal,* or you add your morning latte back in, or whatever it is. And this is where you start to slip back into the habits that messed up your metabolism in the first place.

Remember, my goal is for you *not* to have to be on a diet for the rest of your life. My goal is to repair your metabolism so you can eat at a barbecue, a bar mitzvah, a birthday party, and not experience the aggressive weight gain that comes from a slow metabolism. I want you to be able to enjoy your life, know how to rein it in just a little before and after a big event, stay consistent with your exercise, and be okay with those normal life events, like going out to a restaurant or a party.

But it takes 28 days to get you there. That is not negotiable.

So as good as it feels and fun as it is and as much confidence as you may be feeling right now, watch out. Week three is a dangerous week.

"IF-YOU-THINK-I-LOOK-GOOD-NOW . . ." WEEK— WHAT TO EXPECT, WHAT YOU'RE LIKELY TO FEEL

Obviously, you want to lose weight. The Fast Metabolism Diet will get you there. But what you really need to understand right now, this week, is that weight loss *is not my main goal for you.* I am more vested in giving you a fast, healthy, and optimally functioning metabolism than I am in your losing weight. I'm interested in your finding a weight and place of balance where you can eat and live healthfully every day. Where you can have a full, rich life and not have to diet all the time. If you've already lost a lot of weight, that's awesome, but that doesn't mean your metabolism is fully repaired. I'm not finished with you yet.

Two things happen on the Fast Metabolism Diet: we repair your metabolism, and we give you a fast metabolism. These may both happen quickly, or the repair might take a little longer, before the fast metabolism really kicks in.

This delayed repair often kicks in during week three. I find this happens in particular with clients who have been on low-carb diets for a long time. I had one client who had not eaten any fruit or grain for years. She hadn't even touched brown rice. All she ate was meat, chicken, fish, and vegetables. When she first came to see me, she was very concerned. She told me there was no way she could eat these foods. She said, "If I even look at a piece of toast, I gain three pounds." Her experience is actually not far from what happens to many who have been on low-carb diets for way too long. They become carb-intolerant and really do gain weight with even a small amount of carbohydrates.

In the first two weeks, her weight loss was minimal, and she was very worried. However, I pointed out to her that she was eating hundreds of grams of carbs, *not gaining weight*. This was the repair stage. Her body was relearning how to use the nutrients in carbohydrate-rich foods. After her body learned how to eat carbs again, the weight loss started in earnest, but before her metabolism could begin to burn at a fast rate, she had to repair what she had done with years of low-carb eating.

If, in the first two weeks, you haven't lost as much weight as you had hoped, just notice how many wonderful nutrient-dense carbs you've been eating, and how much healthy fat. When you are holding steady you are also experiencing major metabolism repair. And when the weight loss starts? You've not only repaired your metabolism, but sped it up dramatically. You've not only learned to burn what you eat, but to incinerate your fat stores.

Metabolism repair isn't about losing weight, even though weight loss will happen if you are carrying too much weight for your body. It's about your body being able to extract the nutrients from your food effectively and thoroughly, so you can have the normal and proper biochemical and physiological responses to life. Important things like a healthy release of sex hormones, good skin and hair and nails, sharp brain function, prevention of diseases such as diabetes, heart disease, stroke, and breast cancer. Weight loss is just another pleasant side effect to having a fast metabolism.

There is a larger picture here. Celebrate your success, but don't pat yourself on the back so hard that you knock yourself over. Don't celebrate by going off the program *before* you've completed the entire healing cycle. There are plenty of other nonfood ways to celebrate, like eyeballing some new clothes or treating yourself to a body scrub, facial or pedicure, or even planning a yoga retreat or a health and wellness retreat for when you've finished the 28 days.

This is so crucial, and I can't emphasize this enough: If you cheat now, if you stop now, *all you are doing is repeating old patterns and sticking to the same tired paradigm.* You remember the one. It's the one you used to live by, the prison I'm trying to break you out of. It's the thinking that, "I will always be on some diet," or "I have to go on a diet to get into these clothes or go to that event." It's the old paradigm of, "I can't take it anymore because my weight has gotten out of control, and I'm so dissatisfied with my body that I'll put myself through anything." Remember?

I don't want you to have to feel like that ever again. That's the whole point of metabolism repair. When your metabolism is on fire, then you'll always be able to get into those clothes or go to that event. I don't want you to ever have to feel like your weight has gotten out of control. I don't want you to be dissatisfied with your body. I want you to eat *like a normal person.* This isn't temporary weight loss. All the way through this program, you are learning to reset your metabolism through eating, rather than depressing your metabolism through dieting. By now you are in full swing, in the middle of a biochemical, neurochemical, and physiological transformation that will yield you a killer metabolism.

Sometimes, my clients are tempted to stop the diet during this week. It's so crucial *not* to do this! You absolutely must do the 28 days the first time through. Later, you can revisit the diet for maintenance, and do just a week or two at a time. That's no problem at all. Many of my clients do the Fast Metabolism Diet quarterly, to tease and entice the body so it will continue to have a fast speedy metabolism. This seasonal stoking of the metabolic fire enriches the body, stimulates absorption of nutrients, and reminds the body to transform those nutrients into the right kinds of substances and structures, like muscles, bones, hormones, and feel-good brain chemistry. Some of my clients do it just once or twice a year, to remind them of what a healthy, well-balanced nutritional program looks like. These are amazing and impactful ideas my clients have come up with, but you are on the full 28 day plan right now, so you *must stick to it!*

I help clients get ready for NBA playoff games, red-carpet reveals, and grueling concert tours. I insist they stick to my plan until showtime.

It's more important than ever to be diligent as the healing of your metabolism progresses. I am not ready to turn you loose to show off that body. It isn't your showtime yet. Showtime is 28 days from the day you began the Fast Metabolism Diet. This is not only your rehabilitation and repair but also your final push to achieve that ultimate burn. If you go off the program now, your body will have only experienced the three phases during two weeks of your monthly 28-day cycle.

Your body hasn't run through the entire repair cycle yet. Do you take your clothes out of the washing machine before the rinse cycle? Do you drive your car away from the shop halfway through the oil change? Do you sit up in the middle of emergency surgery and say, "Okay, Doc, I think that's enough for today."

When I was younger, I got into a serious, life-threatening auto accident. I had to do years of physical therapy, occupational therapy, and speech therapy. It was grueling and difficult, but I had a really good surgeon who was passionate about my understanding the big picture. He had honorary Super Bowl rings because of the miraculous work he did rehabilitating NFL players, as well as professional golf and hockey players. He would always tell me, "We'll know we've had success when you're back on the field." That was the motto in the office. So I visualized myself as an athlete who had to get back into the game. The point of physical therapy wasn't just to improve my range of motion, but to have me really be back on top again.

The Fast Metabolism Diet is the same. It's not just about the weight loss. It's about eating again and having your body perform metabolically like a professional's. Its aim is to get you back into the game of life and out of the isolation of dieting.

Like me, this doctor was a drill sergeant. It was his way or the highway, he explained. I had to be consistent. I had to be steady. I had to be diligent. I had to show up, or he wouldn't treat me. I had to work his whole program until he was ready to discharge me.

I'm not ready to discharge you. You will be discharged after 28 days, no sooner. So as good as you look now, as good as you *would* look with a drink in your hand, hold off on that drink for a little bit longer. Don't check out yet, because you are *not done*.

This program is not a quick fix. Week three is crucial, so stay focused, stay steady, and keep your eye on the prize of having a fast metabolism and never depriving yourself of eating real food again.

DON'T LET EXERCISE SLIDE THIS WEEK!

Don't forget to continue with your phase-appropriate exercise: one or two days of moderate cardio during Phase 1, one or two days of heavy weight lifting during Phase 2, and one to three days of ultra-relaxing activity in Phase 3. This is no time to let exercise slide. You are releasing fat at a rapid rate by now, and your body is working diligently to convert that fat to fuel. You do not want to redeposit it to another place in your body. You want to burn it up or convert it into muscle by exercising! Remember to keep your exercise *strictly phase-specific* for 28 days. This is a must for true structural transformation.

You have to move to build muscle. Use your new energy and confidence to step it up a little within each phase. You're getting faster, stronger, and better at relaxing, so embrace what's happening. Your body is transforming before your eyes.

WHAT TO EAT: YOUR DAILY MEAL MAP FOR WEEK THREE

Once again, I've provided you with a meal map that tells you exactly what to eat within this week. Remember, you can switch meals within phases, or use some of the meals I suggest, but not others. If you want to eat leftovers from week one all week long and not cook at all, great. If you want to try all new dishes, great. As long as you are sticking to the phase-specific foods at each meal and snack and your portions are correct, you can adapt this plan to your own needs.

Now is also a good time to reread the Fast Metabolism Rules (page 85). Don't you dare start phase-swapping! You look good, but you do not yet get to eat like you have a fast metabolism.

148   THE FAST METABOLISM DIET

I have a client named Layla, who lost a lot of weight on the Fast Metabolism Diet, but not during week three. Instead, she gained weight, for the exact reason I warn you about—she was looking good and she knew it! She felt that she was out of crisis. And, she was crazy busy. So she cheated a little here, a little there, let up on the water, had some wine, a little dessert. She also skipped lunch on Monday and then had cheesecake for dinner. She reduced the fruit in her Phase 1 lunches to compensate (which doesn't work), and she had lamb during Phase 2, which is only on the Phase 3 list. Her weight loss stalled and she even gained a pound on one day.

Layla wasn't ready yet. Her metabolism was improving, but it wasn't fully repaired. Though she was having an especially busy week, letting up on water is a big mistake. Water is crucial in flushing out toxins that are getting released from all the fat you are burning. If you reduce water in this week, your adrenal hormones will signal the body to slow weight loss while it plays catchup with the toxins you are releasing. You also have to stay within the phases until the 28 days are over, and don't eat more and don't eat less. Don't skip meal or snack times. Don't eat out of phase until your body is ready—and it isn't ready yet. Not to worry, she got right back on track and shed her guilt so she could shed her pounds—and she looks hot! It just took her a little longer to get to where she wanted to be.

Stay strong because you're looking great! Just one more week to go. The last week is easy. You're becoming a pro at this Fast Metabolism thing. The weight is continuing to fall off, so stay with the plan and keep up the great work.

You're doing it. I can just imagine you now. You're probably out there beginning to coach your friends and coworkers, showing off your lunches and snacks with pride. You're no longer hiding and isolated in the world of dieting. You are a bit of a foodie and getting excited about all that food can do for your body. It's happening. You're becoming one of those people. You know which ones I'm talking about, the ones who declare, "Oh, I just have a fast metabolism."

WEEK THREE MEAL MAP, *PHASE 1*

PHASE 1: UNWIND STRESS

	WAKE TIME	WEIGHT	BREAKFAST	SNACK	LUNCH	SNACK	DINNER	EXERCISE	WATER
MONDAY	__:__ am/pm	____	__:__ am/pm P1 FROZEN MANGO FAT-BURNING SMOOTHIE	__:__ am/pm 1 ORANGE	__:__ am/pm P1 TUNA, GREEN APPLE, AND SPINACH SALAD 10 RICE CRACKERS	__:__ am/pm 1 CUP POMEGRANATE SEEDS	__:__ am/pm P1 ITALIAN CHICKEN AND WILD RICE		
TUESDAY	__:__ am/pm	____	__:__ am/pm P1 OATMEAL	__:__ am/pm 1 CUP FROZEN PINEAPPLE	__:__ am/pm P1 ITALIAN CHICKEN AND WILD RICE (LEFTOVER) 1 CUP PAPAYA	__:__ am/pm 1 ORANGE	__:__ am/pm P1 TURKEY CHILI		

WEEK THREE MEAL MAP, *PHASE 2*

				PHASE 2: UNLOCK FAT				
WAKE TIME	WEIGHT	BREAKFAST	SNACK	LUNCH	SNACK	DINNER	EXERCISE	WATER
WEDNESDAY ___:___ am/pm	_____	___:___ am/pm P2 SPANISH EGG WHITE SCRAMBLE	___:___ am/pm TURKEY JERKY	___:___ am/pm P2 ROAST BEEF, MUSTARD, AND LETTUCE WRAP	___:___ am/pm ½ PORTION P2 TUNA AND CUCUMBER SALAD	___:___ am/pm P2 BROILED HALIBUT WITH BROCCOLI		
THURSDAY ___:___ am/pm	_____	___:___ am/pm P2 EGG WHITE, MUSHROOM, AND SPINACH OMELET	___:___ am/pm ½ PORTION (LEFTOVER) P2 TUNA AND CUCUMBER SALAD	___:___ am/pm SPINACH SALAD WITH LEFTOVER HALIBUT, WITH CILANTRO AND LIME JUICE	___:___ am/pm ROAST BEEF SLICES AND CUCUMBER SLICES	___:___ am/pm P2 PEPPERONCINI PORK ROAST		

WEEK THREE MEAL MAP, *PHASE 3*

PHASE 3: UNLEASH YOUR METABOLISM

	WAKE TIME	WEIGHT	BREAKFAST	SNACK	LUNCH	SNACK	DINNER	EXERCISE	WATER
FRIDAY	___:___ am/pm	____	___:___ am/pm SPROUTED TOAST WITH NUT BUTTER AND BERRIES P3 VEGGIE	___:___ am/pm 2 OUNCES SHRIMP WITH LEMON WEDGES	___:___ am/pm P3 THREE-EGG SALAD WITH TOMATOES, RASPBERRIES	___:___ am/pm ¼ CUP RAW ALMONDS	___:___ am/pm P3 SHRIMP AND VEGGIE STIR-FRY		
SATURDAY	___:___ am/pm		___:___ am/pm P3 BERRY NUTTY OATMEAL SMOOTHIE P3 VEGGIE	___:___ am/pm ½ AVOCADO WITH SEA SALT	___:___ am/pm P3 ENDIVE TUNA SALAD, PEACH	___:___ am/pm P3 THREE-EGG SALAD ½ PORTION	___:___ am/pm P3 COCONUT CURRY CHICKEN		
SUNDAY	___:___ am/pm		___:___ am/pm P3 THREE-EGG SALAD (LEFTOVER) ON SPROUTED GRAIN TORTILLA 1 PEACH	___:___ am/pm CELERY WITH ALMOND BUTTER AND CAROB CHIPS	___:___ am/pm P3 COCONUT CURRY CHICKEN (LEFTOVER)	___:___ am/pm ¼ CUP RAW ALMONDS	___:___ am/pm P3 SESAME CHICKEN STIR-FRY		

CHAPTER NINE

Week Four: Give It Hell

I'm so proud of you. Here you are in week four. By now, you have likely begun not just to eat in an entirely new way, but to think about food in a new way, as well. For many, this will have been a big transition. You've done it! Here you are, in the very last week.

This is the week to look back at what you've done for the past 21 days. Whether you've built your own maps or followed the menus I've created, pull them out and look at what worked for you. Did you increase your spinach and broccoli portions in Phase 2, and did that seem to help you fill up and lose more weight? Did you notice that the French toast in Phase 1 made you feel more satisfied than plain toast with fruit? Did you notice that oatmeal or chili in particular made you feel warm and fuzzy?

What are the keys that have led to your success so far? Let this be your week to contemplate the things that you loved, that really lowered your stress hormones, and that made you feel great.

Then give it hell.

This is the week to really do it. Be perfect. Be strong. Be awesome. Hit every phase exactly right. Do every phase-appropriate exercise. Complete the repair process and light that metabolism on fire.

This is also a good week to do everything you've wanted to do during the four weeks that you haven't done yet: look through the recipe chapter for those you didn't get to try yet. Make them! (Or, stick to your favorites or leftovers from past weeks, if that's easier.) If there are phase-appropriate exercises you still haven't tried yet (A meditation class? A deep breathing seminar in person or online?), go for it! Generally, my clients tell me they have a pretty easy time with week four. They realize they are coming to the end, they feel good about their weight loss, and they want to finish strong.

So do it! You have been using food as medicine to enhance your health and well-being, so you should be feeling really good—balanced and stable, in control of your cravings, stronger and lighter and better than you did four weeks ago. Make this last week the best week ever, and really enjoy the incredible job you have done.

GIVE-IT-HELL WEEK—WHAT TO EXPECT, WHAT YOU'RE LIKELY TO FEEL

You're entering the last week of your personal four-week cycle, and the last week of the Fast Metabolism Diet. Remember, your body, in this particular part of its own four-week cycle, has *never experienced this particular diet.* To your body, each of the four weeks is an entirely new experience because you are in a different place metabolically. You are at different stages of repair and rebuilding, and each time you experience each of the three phases, you bring a healthier body to the table. But even if you are happy with your weight-loss number, you still have to remember that your body isn't completely repaired yet. You're so close, but you don't want to stop before you reach the finish line.

Really drive home the principles this week. Stick precisely and exactly to the meal map and the grocery list, even if you dream about having a glass of wine or a dessert next week. This is the final week to stoke your metabolism. No more damp logs!

GIVE IT HELL

Exercise is like lighter fluid for your metabolic fire. Exercise is the difference between starting a fire with a match and starting a fire with a match and lighter fluid. We've all seen the dramatic results you get with that extra boost that takes your spark and makes it burn. So give it hell—one or two days of moderate cardio during Phase 1, one or two days of heavy weight lifting during Phase 2, and one to three days of ultra-relaxing activity in Phase 3, like yoga, a walk outdoors on a nice day, or a massage. Think about whether you would like to maintain this schedule even after the Fast Metabolism Diet is over. A little cardio, a little weight training, and a little stress maintenance every week is crucial to staying healthy. I tell my clients all the time that if I could bottle a product that would give them the same health benefits that moderate exercise and stress reduction give them, I would be a billionaire and we would all be kicking it back on my yacht.

WHAT TO EAT—YOUR MEAL MAP FOR WEEK FOUR

You're going to miss my telling you what to do once these four weeks are over, aren't you? So, one last time, here I go telling you exactly what to eat. Remember that you can switch meals within phases, or use some of the meals I suggest but not others. And remember, you are in the home stretch! This is not the time to get creative with the rules or start phase-swapping. Yes, I did once saw a cast off my ankle a week ahead of time, but I had a very important horse show, I was young, and my mother was working that night, so she wasn't there to tell me not to do it. Let's collectively agree that we are not that young, nor are we stupid, and I am here to prohibit you from straying. You and I both know you need this, you want this, you deserve this. So do not break my rules. Instead, give it hell and finish strong. While you're in the process of following this last week, I want you to start thinking about what's going to happen when the diet is over. I'll talk in more detail about this in Chapter Ten, "Fast Metabolism Living," but by about Wednesday of this last week, you may be thinking: "Wait, what am I going to do next week? This is the end!" This can be a major transition, so while you are in the throes of week four, I want you to be game-planning for your future.

Although some aspects of the metabolism may have a genetic component, in most cases a slow metabolism is due to how you have been living. So how were you living before? How was it different from the way you have been living the last 28 days? What have you learned during the past four weeks about how your body really *wants* to live? What creates an optimal environment for your body, your metabolism, and your overall well-being?

If you feel better, clearer, and more energetic off caffeine, do you really want to go back on it? If you feel happier, calmer, and cleaner without eating refined sugar or gluten or corn, do you really want to go back to eating those things again?

If you do, your metabolism will be better able to handle those foods occasionally, in moderate amounts. But consider how well you are doing without them. Some people *will* go back to unhealthy habits, and a fast metabolism can make up for a lot. But at some point, if you really drag yourself back down again with foods that don't give your body the nutrition it needs, and with foods that contain toxic things it doesn't need that tax your liver and promote fat accumulation, then guess what? You may eventually find yourself back where you started. A fast metabolism is meant to support a healthy lifestyle, not miraculously nullify a totally dysfunctional one.

So this week, as you are giving your all to the plan, think about how you can give your all to your life. And by that, I mean live like you mean it, with purpose and discernment. Take care of your body. You fixed it. Do you really want to break it again?

When you are back to your "normal" life eating like a "normal" person, you have to understand what that means. In case you still aren't sure, look at how you've been eating the past four weeks: You haven't been abstaining from any food group. You've been eating proteins, fruits, vegetables, and grains. You've been losing excess weight steadily. You've been improving your physiology and internal chemistry. You look better. You've been exercising moderately. Your mood has improved. Isn't this how you would like to live all the time?

My goal for you is to learn to live with balance, enjoying your life but not at the expense of your health. Obesity and weight gain cause significant increases in diabetes, breast cancer, depression, heart disease, and many other chronic illnesses. You've set yourself on the right track, and you've been learning what promotes health. You've been participating in it, succeeding in it, making an impact on the scale, your health, your whole life.

I was meeting with a client the other day whom I hadn't seen in years. She was now in the throes of menopause and looking for some natural therapies to help ease her through this hormone transition. She had already put herself back on the Fast Metabolism Diet and had just completed a full 28 days, getting her back to her target weight. She had done a version of the program with me six years earlier, and it was amazing to me how she hadn't forgotten the rhythm and the foods and the phases after all this time. She told me that many of the lifestyle changes from the diet she had maintained as part of her healthy life, but that she felt that she needed a strict tune-up, not only to get back to her ideal weight but also to remind herself how amazing her body felt and responded to being treated so well. She recited to me what she called "Haylie-isms," such as: "Don't fast before going fast" (eat before working out), or "If it's fake, take a break" (no artificial sweeteners), or "If it says free on the label, don't buy it" (no fat-free or sugar-free diet products). I was proud! Proud of her for taking a preventative approach to her health, proud of her for taking the initiative to put herself back on a program that would promote health and allow her to achieve an ideal body weight, and proud that she had taken me and my dorky little sayings with her on her life's journeys for the past six years.

So as we spend this last week together of this short 28-day program, think about keeping me as your nutritionist for many more years. I'm with you for life—and you can enjoy the rest of it in better health, better balance, and at the healthiest possible weight.

Think about making healthy, balanced food choices from now on. Think about preferring nutrient-dense over nutrient-poor foods most of the time. Think about moving and practicing stress relief and eating tons of vegetables. Think about everything you've learned, and think about how you can live it, this week, next week, and for the rest of your life. Take all that you've gleaned forward with you. You know how to stimulate the five major players. You have the tools to ignite, stoke, entice, and keep your metabolism going, so during this week embrace the changes you have made and look at how some of them can be not just life changing but also changes for life.

WEEK FOUR MEAL MAP, PHASE 1

PHASE 1: UNWIND STRESS

WAKE TIME	WEIGHT	BREAKFAST	SNACK	LUNCH	SNACK	DINNER	EXERCISE	WATER
MONDAY __:__ am/pm	____	__:__ am/pm P1 FROZEN MANGO FAT-BURNING SMOOTHIE	__:__ am/pm 1 APPLE	__:__ am/pm P1 OPEN-FACED TURKEY SANDWICH, FIGS	__:__ am/pm 1 CUP FROZEN PINEAPPLE	__:__ am/pm P1 TURKEY, WHITE BEAN, AND KALE SOUP		
TUESDAY __:__ am/pm	____	__:__ am/pm P1 STRAWBERRY FRENCH TOAST	__:__ am/pm 1 ORANGE	__:__ am/pm P1 TURKEY, WHITE BEAN, AND KALE SOUP (LEFTOVER), SLICED MANGO	__:__ am/pm 1 ASIAN PEAR	__:__ am/pm P1 ITALIAN CHICKEN AND WILD RICE		

WEEK FOUR MEAL MAP, PHASE 2

PHASE 2: UNLOCK FAT

WAKE TIME	WEIGHT	BREAKFAST	SNACK	LUNCH	SNACK	DINNER	EXERCISE	WATER
__:__ am/pm **WEDNESDAY**		__:__ am/pm P2 EGG WHITE, MUSHROOM, AND SPINACH OMELET	__:__ am/pm TURKEY SLICES AND MUSTARD	__:__ am/pm P1 2 CUPS BEEF, KALE, AND LEEK SOUP	__:__ am/pm TURKEY JERKY	__:__ am/pm P2 BAKED CINNAMON-MUSTARD CHICKEN AND LEMON-GARLIC SPINACH		
__:__ am/pm **THURSDAY**		__:__ am/pm P2 SMOKED SALMON AND CUCUMBERS	__:__ am/pm 3 HARD-BOILED EGG WHITES WITH SEA SALT	__:__ am/pm P2 BAKED CINNAMON-MUSTARD CHICKEN (LEFTOVER) ON SALAD WITH P2 SALAD DRESSING	__:__ am/pm TURKEY SLICES AND MUSTARD	__:__ am/pm P2 BEEF, KALE, AND LEEK SOUP (LEFTOVER)		

WEEK FOUR MEAL MAP, *PHASE 3*

PHASE 3: UNLEASH YOUR METABOLISM

WAKE TIME	WEIGHT	BREAKFAST	SNACK	LUNCH	SNACK	DINNER	EXERCISE	WATER
FRIDAY ___:___ am/pm	____	___:___ am/pm 1 SLICE SPROUTED-GRAIN TOAST WITH ½ AVOCADO, TOMATO SLICE, AND CUCUMBER SLICES	___:___ am/pm 2 OUNCES SHRIMP WITH LEMON WEDGES	___:___ am/pm P3 OLIVE AND TOMATO SALAD WITH CHICKEN OR TURKEY SLICES	___:___ am/pm RED BELL PEPPER STRIPS DIPPED IN P3 SALAD DRESSING	___:___ am/pm P3 SESAME CHICKEN STIR-FRY		
SATURDAY ___:___ am/pm	____	___:___ am/pm P3 BERRY NUTTY OATMEAL SMOOTHIE P3 VEGGIE	___:___ am/pm ½ AVOCADO WITH SEA SALT	___:___ am/pm P3 ENDIVE TUNA SALAD, APPLE	___:___ am/pm CELERY AND HUMMUS	___:___ am/pm P3 ROSEMARY PORK ROAST WITH SWEET POTATO		
SUNDAY ___:___ am/pm	____	___:___ am/pm CELERY WITH ALMOND BUTTER AND CAROB CHIPS, CHERRIES, 2 RICE CRACKERS	___:___ am/pm CELERY WITH P3 DIP OR SALAD DRESSING	___:___ am/pm SALAD WITH 2 CUPS SPINACH, ⅓ CUP HUMMUS, CHERRY TOMATOES, CELERY, CILANTRO, AND P3 SALAD DRESSING	___:___ am/pm ¼ CUP RAW ALMONDS	___:___ am/pm P3 AVOCADO QUESADILLA, SIDE MIXED GREENS WITH P3 DRESSING		

You might want to take one last freezer, fridge, and pantry inventory, and switch out any of these meals with foods you already have on hand. Then finish out the week with your favorites from the past weeks, or the recipes from the recipe chapter that you've been dying to try. And if you don't get to try everything, don't worry; these are recipes you can continue to make and enjoy after the Fast Metabolism Diet is over. My kids each have their favorite meals from the recipe chapter, and I use many of the recipes for entertaining, so these are not just recipes for "a diet." They are recipes for life.

You're done! You did it! When you get to the end of this week and you've lost even half a pound a day through the whole four weeks, you have completely rehabilitated your dysfunctional metabolism, creating an abundance of health, balanced hormones, stabilized cholesterol, and healthy immune system production. We've done a lot of work together these last 28 days—you, me, and the five major players. I am very proud of you and I look forward to working together on other life ventures. Before I cut you loose, though, I want to talk about living with your new, beautiful, to-be-cherished body.

Part IV:
Fast
Metabolism
in Action

CHAPTER TEN

HAYLIE
POMROY

Fast Metabolism Living

Congratulations! You've just done something incredible. You've re-paired your metabolism, lit it on fire, and burned through fat like never before. And you did it with everything you've been afraid of in the past. You did it by enjoying food. No drugs, no surgery, no torture. Just real, delicious food, coupled with an easy amount of physical activity and some critical stress reduction. You should be feeling amazing, and much different than you did before you began.

Let's check in with where you are. I bet you're feeling much different from how you did before you began because your liver, adrenals, thyroid, pituitary, and physical body are finally getting everything they really need. Take a look in the mirror. Does your skin look better and more supple? Is your body more toned? Is your hair thicker, shinier, healthier? Are your nails growing faster? Do you have more energy? How many inches did you lose? How many pounds? Do your clothes fit differently?

I want you to think about how your life has changed these past four weeks. What have you loved about following this way of eating? Did you enjoy coming home and savoring the aroma of food cooking in the slow cooker? How did you feel after eating mangos at 4:00 P.M. in the afternoon, instead of some fake sugary snack? What was it like to have a healthy lunch all packed and ready to go every morning, and a freezer pregnant with de-licious options for dinner?

What was life like having breakfast every day, and never going to bed hungry? How did it feel to have your family drift into the kitchen when they smelled something delicious and healthy cooking? Did you like being able to eat with friends and even entertain while on this diet? Did you like having such a clear system for how to eat? Think about all the experiences you've had in the last four weeks. What things would you like to keep doing in your daily life?

But are you ready for regular life yet?

You've completed 28 days, but have you reached your weight goal? Turn back to page 104, where you wrote down the weight you want to be. How close are you?

If you had much more than 20 pounds to lose, you probably aren't there yet. But don't worry. If you still have more weight to lose, you can simply do the plan again. In fact, you can do this program forever and thrive. Whether you need to lose another 20 pounds or 40 or even 100, you can eat your way to your goal weight, and to sustained, lasting health.

REPEATING THE DIET

If you still have weight to lose, I recommend turning right around and repeating the 28-day cycle again. Many of my clients follow up with two or three cycles of the diet, until they get to where they want to be. But, what if you have just another 5, 7, or 10 pounds to lose?

Not a problem. After you've done the first four weeks, you can do as many additional weeks as you need—one, two, seven, whatever—until you reach the weight you want to be. Even if you are just a few pounds away from your ideal weight, even fewer than 5 pounds away, keep going until you reach it. It may only take an additional week or two, but do it. Get there. Otherwise, I guarantee you that in five years, you're still going to be messing around with those same 5 pounds. Just get rid of them now, and let someone else tell that story of how close they got to their goals . . . you'll have achieved yours.

As I said earlier, many of my clients love to do the 28 days every quarter, just to keep the metabolism trained, like an athlete. Others do it once or twice a year. I have one client who did two full rounds of the Fast Metabolism Diet and achieved her goal weight in those first 56 days. However, she lives a very hectic and demanding lifestyle and travels all the time, so she does one week of the Fast Metabolism Diet on the first week of every month. She has done this religiously for years, and it works for her. She says it keeps her metabolism on fire and the glow lasts all month long. She says it also reminds her that she can actually cook nourishing, comforting, enriching food, and those domestic goddess moments keep her grounded.

Whether you do the Fast Metabolism Diet for 28 days or another four, six, or eight cycles, at some point, you'll need to stop the weight loss and settle in at a happy, healthy weight. I have a few rules, shocking I know, for when you get there.

When you are at your goal weight, you have graduated from dieting. You've tasted true, vibrant health, and this chapter is going to show you how to continue to reap all the healthy benefits you've worked so hard to achieve. This is a maintenance plan that really works, and works for life.

RULES FOR MAINTENANCE

1. If It's Fake, Huge Mistake
2. Always Eat Within 30 Minutes of Waking
3. Don't Fast Before Going Fast
4. Three Meals, Two Snacks
5. Celebrate the Seasons
6. Embrace Your Culture
7. Make Time and Cupcakes
8. Chart Your Path
9. Keep Cooking and Slow Cooking
10. Keep Freezing
11. Maintain Your Crash Stash
12. Stay Quit
13. Drink Up
14. Keep Moving
15. Repeat the Diet as Needed
16. Stay Organic
17. Supplement
18. Chill Out
19. Keep Loving Food

HEALTHY LIVING FOR A LIFETIME

I love my horses. I feed them well, groom them well, and indulge them. They get a lot of attention, but that's nothing compared to the way some of the great racehorses and performance horses get treated, with private masseuses soothing their muscles, Reiki masters manipulating their energy, and horse blankets with magnets sewn into them to treat inflammation. They eat six meals a day and get multiple grooming sessions. They are pampered and cherished. You can spot the horses who are fed really well. When they are performing, they shine, radiating beauty and confidence.

Why don't you treat yourself this way? You can! Now that you've given your metabolism a wake-up call and coaxed it back into shape, I want you to see yourself the way a trainer would see a valuable performance horse. I want you to value yourself and respect and nourish yourself so that you can stay at the top of your game. I want you to glow. Let life be your performance ring. Treat yourself like you've got the potential to win the Triple Crown. Shake your mane and step out into the world. I want you to respect your own level of metabolic performance. Cherish what you've accomplished in your own body. Move forward into your future with pride and dignity and a commitment never to abuse your body again.

You are a champion. You have been in my stable, and you will now reflect the care you have given yourself the past 28 days.

This level of self-care should be your new reality, as you step back into real life after 28 days on the Fast Metabolism Diet. I know that right now you might be feeling a little nervous. Going back to real life can feel a little scary. What if you go back to all your old, bad habits?

Don't worry. You have formed so many good ones here that they don't stand a chance. Plus, you're stronger than you were a month ago.

But in order to maintain your weight loss by maintaining your fast metabolism, there are some critical principles that I recommend to follow in your regular life.

THE FAST METABOLISM TOOLS FOR LIFE

TOOL #1. IF IT'S FAKE, HUGE MISTAKE.

No matter what you eat, make sure it's real food. People are so obsessed with reading labels and counting calories or carbs or fat grams, but I say, screw that! Look at the ingredients list. If you don't know what every ingredient is, then put it down. A little raw sugar, some vegetable oil, those things are okay. At least you know what they are. But if you don't know what it is, leave it on the shelf. In particular, watch out for fake sugars and fake fats. These are huge metabolism killers and they are not real food.

TOOL #2. ALWAYS EAT WITHIN 30 MINUTES OF WAKING.

Grandma always says breakfast is the most important meal of the day. This is a good habit for life. If you don't eat right after you wake up in the morning, you are requiring your body to think, work, drive, and do everything else you need to do in your day on zero fuel. In response, your adrenals will produce that emergency hormone that tells your body it had better start stockpiling fat because who knows when you'll get more food. We've worked so hard to transform your fat into muscle during this program, and this is no time to mess that up. Keep the muscle, lose the fat: Eat breakfast!

TOOL #3. DON'T FAST BEFORE GOING FAST.

Never get up and exercise in the morning before you've eaten breakfast or at least a snack. Eat at least 30 minutes before exercising. Otherwise, your adrenals will stimulate a hormone to break down muscle for fuel during your workout, cannibalizing the muscles you're trying to build. What a waste of a workout! A piece of fruit is the ideal pre-workout snack. Then have a snack containing 10 to 20 grams of protein afterwards. That will set you up perfectly to get the most from your workout. The natural sugars in the fruit fuel the muscle motion during the workout, and the protein aids in rapid repair. This is an ideal formula for fat burning and muscle building so you continue to sculpt and develop a healthy physique.

TOOL #4. THREE MEALS, TWO SNACKS.

Stay in the habit of eating three meals and two snacks every single day. This will keep your metabolism stoked and burning through the food you eat. Don't forget to plant Crash Stashes at home, at work, in your car, at the gym, etc. (The recipe chapter includes a great list of Crash Stash snacks you can enjoy both on and off the diet.) Although you aren't eating in phases anymore, I recommend keeping some type of phase rotation when it comes to snacks. Two days of fruit snacks, two days of protein snacks, and three days of healthy fat-based snacks will keep you out of a rut and keep your metabolism guessing. This helps to ensure your body will never become resistant to any type of foods, and it sets you up for rapid burn if garbage (like that ice cream you've been dreaming about) ever happens to pass your lips (only to be consumed by your roaring metabolic fire).

TOOL #5. CELEBRATE THE SEASONS.

Study after study shows that the body's digestion, hormonal output, and structure changes with the seasons. Nature mirrors this in its production of different foods at different times of the year. Eating seasonal foods—like watermelon and berries in the summer, apples in the fall, and root vegetables in the winter—help to support the body's natural rhythm and its connection with nature. Typically this is also a more affordable way of eating, as well celebrating food and boosting those feel-good, metabolism-enhancing hormones.

TOOL #6. EMBRACE YOUR CULTURE.

Chinese New Year, Day of the Dead, Christmas, Thanksgiving, Hanukkah, Kwanza or any other religious or cultural-based holiday, seem to always have a major food component. Embrace this, celebrate this, and make coming together to share food and tradition a good thing. For some, family time can bring about unique stressors. Often we let one holiday celebration bleed into the next, losing the specialness of a moment and instead falling into a downward spiral of gluttony. This stress topped with overindulgence is a recipe for disaster. Instead, learn new recipes from your elders and enjoy the meaning of the event but do not allow it to destroy your healthy path to a Fast Metabolism lifestyle.

TOOL #7. MAKE TIME AND CUPCAKES.

I have a motto: If I bake it then my metabolism can take it! But if I'm going to splurge, it's not going to be mindless munching on packaged junk food, so if I didn't take the time to bake it then we try to not have that dessert in our home. So that means we have to go out for ice cream or frozen yogurt, and I don't keep packaged cookies, cakes, or pies in the house. I feel that what we bake in our home is healthier, made with love, and metabolizes faster. It also takes effort and intention and gives me time to think if maybe I am just stressed, thirsty, or truly hungry and that is why I am having sugar cravings. This is another healthy way I try to get in touch with the food I eat.

TOOL #8. CHART YOUR PATH.

Sit down on the weekend and plan your week ahead of time. Chart out at least your dinners, breakfast, and snacks. I do this with clients all day long and the comment I get again and again is that this makes their lives so much easier. I have a method in our busy home. I use a crockpot and make a soup each weekend. This gets us through four dinners and two lunches. I sometimes convert the chicken from a soup to a salad or burrito for the next day's lunch. We have smoothies for breakfast twice a week and a loaded hot cereal twice a week, and eggs and bacon or avocado and toast or Greek yogurt to round out the last three breakfasts. These are just a given and so routine I literally can pull this off in my sleep. For the remaining three dinners, we grill once, eat out once, and one night is "fend for yourself" night in our household just so no one forgets to appreciate me! It works with my busy lifestyle and keeps me fueled for all I am trying to pull off.

TOOL #9. KEEP COOKING AND SLOW COOKING.

When you're too busy to cook, get the slow cooker ready the night before and put the "bowl" in the fridge. In the morning, plug it in, turn it on, and go. You'll come home to a hot dinner so delicious you won't even be tempted by frozen dinners or takeout. Keep making the recipes you loved from the book, and go ahead and make the recipes you didn't get to try. Just because the 28 days is over that doesn't mean you can't keep making the recipes! I frequently make these recipes for my family, I serve them at dinner parties, I take them to potlucks, and I keep them in the freezer for everyone's lunches and dinners. For hundreds more recipes that fit the plan or your newly healthy lifestyle, look for the Fast Metabolism Cookbook coming out soon, or visit my website: www.fastmetabolismdiet.com.

TOOL #10. KEEP FREEZING.

As you've probably noticed by now, my freezer gets a lot of use. I cook up fruit and freeze it so I always have a topping for French toast. Whenever I chop up veggies, I chop extra and put them in the freezer for those days when I don't have time for chopping. When you always have food pre-made, it's so easy to make a quick meal! At the end of each week, continue to do your freezer inventory. See what you have left over, and use those things the next week, so nothing gets wasted.

TOOL #11. MAINTAIN YOUR CRASH STASH.

You should always, always have a Crash Stash snack in your purse, your car, your office, and your freezer. This way, no matter where you are, if you get hungry or it has been three or four hours since you last ate and you need healthy food fast, you'll be ready. (See list of Crash Stash snacks on page 183.)

TOOL #12. STAY QUIT.

Keep avoiding caffeine, gluten, corn, soy, sugar, alcohol, and processed foods most of the time. Your metabolism can handle the occasional splurge now, such as on special occasions, but you are doing so well, do you really want to go back to mainlining metabolism killers? If you are someone who likes her grains, eat the sprouted-grain or wheat-free varieties. "Enriched" breads and pastas have almost all the nutrients stripped from them, then gluten and chemicals are sprayed on to make them taste good. They are fake foods. See Rule #1.

TOOL #13. DRINK UP.

Keep drinking half your body weight in fluid ounces of water every day. This is an essential life habit that couldn't be easier to follow. When you are dehydrated, you will actually retain water and get that bloated, puffy appearance. Remember, drinking a lot of water flushes waste and toxins from the body, enhancing the metabolism with every sip you take. Spring water is ideal. Sip on it throughout the day instead of trying to catch up at night right before you go to bed.

TOOL #14. KEEP MOVING.

Continue to exercise three times per week every week, rotating burning (cardio), building (weight lifting), and healing exercises (remember massage counts as a healing exercise) just the way you did during the 28 days. You can do more if you want to, but do at least this much. The more active you are, the more mitochondria your cells will have. Remember, the mitochondria are the fat furnaces of the cell!

TOOL #15. REPEAT THE DIET AS NEEDED.

When and if you feel the need to refresh and refuel your metabolism, repeat the Fast Metabolism Diet. Some of my clients do it every quarter, or twice a year, or even annually, to add kindling to the metabolic fire. Once you've done the full 28 days, you can do the whole thing again or you can do just a week or two at some regular interval. Do what keeps you on track. When you do just a week every quarter, your body will remember: *Oh, yes! This is what we do to get me back into shape and feeling awesome!*

If you keep up with maintenance, you won't necessarily have to repeat the Fast Metabolism Diet, but many of my clients choose to do it because they love it, and they enjoy doing it on a certain schedule. It adds structure and a feeling of nurture to their lives. Repeating the diet will ensure that your metabolism can withstand changing life circumstances, such as hormone changes, stress, trauma, the birth of a child, or anything else life throws at you. Think of repeating the Fast Metabolism Diet as like sweeping the patio after a storm. Even after you've cleaned it, the weather can change and you may need to sweep again. Or think of it like this: just because you broke your leg once and repaired it once doesn't mean you will never injure yourself and need repair again. Implement this diet at any time when healing from an injury, targeting weight loss, stabilizing blood sugars, balancing hormones, or reducing cholesterol. Use it when you need it, and keep the awe for what your body can do when you treat it right.

TOOL #16. STAY ORGANIC.

Organic really matters, especially with your dairy, chicken, eggs, and beef. Trust this aggie when I tell you that you do not want what the nonorganic versions of these things have to offer you! Let's just leave it at that.

TOOL #17. SUPPLEMENT.

Because of both poor soil quality and the tendency of most people to at least occasionally make poor food choices, consider covering your nutritional bases with basic supplements, especially a high-quality, clean multi-vitamin and a food-based essential fatty-acid supplement. You may already have your favorite brands, or check out the Fast Metabolism supplements on my website, www.fastmetabolismdiet.com.

TOOL #18. CHILL OUT.

Now you understand how absolutely crucial it is to keep stress at bay, so don't let it get the better of you. Learn to relax, breathe deeply, take care of yourself, and say no when you are overextended. Anything else just isn't worth the metabolic price.

TOOL #19. KEEP LOVING FOOD.

Never stop loving what real, nutrient-dense food does for you and your body. Appreciate and respect what nutrients have to offer and the potential they hold for you. Stay in tune with how you feel before you eat, and how you feel after you eat, to keep tabs on what foods make you feel good and what foods you are better off avoiding. Love healthy fats and complex carbs. You never have to fear food again.

FAST METABOLISM SURVIVAL TIPS—BECAUSE LIFE HAPPENS

You've lost the weight, and it's staying off. You're making good choices and living a happy, healthy, Fast Metabolism life. And then it happens . . . *the event.* The dinner party, the wedding, the birthday, the date at a fancy restaurant. You know you're supposed to be able to eat like a healthy person now, but you're nervous. You want to enjoy yourself and relax, but you find yourself getting stressed because, *What if you blow it?*

If this happens, first remind yourself that you are facing these events as a different person because we've repaired your metabolism and you have so many new tools, like food. Remember, food is your friend now.

Just because you are off the program that doesn't mean everything you've learned in this book has left you. All the resources, knowledge, and habits you've acquired can come with you, through your parties and your events. You're not going to that party alone. Plus, it's especially important to remember that the whole purpose of fixing your metabolism was so you can enjoy the special events in life, indulge a little, and not have to pay some catastrophic price.

But in case you're still worried, I'm going to let you in on a few of my little secrets that can help minimize the damage when you know you're going to splurge. These are the secrets I share with my celebrity clients, who can't afford to look bloated or gain 5 pounds after a night on the town.

SPLURGE SECRET #1: THE BIG DINNER.

Maybe you know you're going to pig out at a Mexican restaurant tonight, or you've got a church potluck that's going to last all weekend, or you're facing a lavish buffet with too many can't-miss items. Whatever it is, you know you're going to be eating a lot. To minimize the damage, all you have to do are two things:

1. EAT 10 TO 15 GRAMS OF PROTEIN *EVERY TWO HOURS* THROUGHOUT THE DAY, from 30 minutes after waking until you arrive at the event. Eat like it's Phase 2—low-glycemic, lots of vegetables, but especially protein, and especially animal protein, which is the most easily absorbed. Have protein-rich meals and between meals, eat slices of chicken breast or nitrate-free turkey deli meat, an ounce or two of leftover steak or pork loin or fish. This will keep your blood sugar stable and your muscles will have fuel to store any extra sugars (like the wine or the margarita you plan to drink) as glycogen instead of fat.

This will also put the brakes on bingeing and out-of-control party eating because you'll show up hungry, but not famished. Finally, eating protein every two hours all day without fail will kick your fat-burning hormones into gear. They'll be primed and pumped to handle anything you shovel in.

2. GET REALLY EXCITED ABOUT THE EVENT. This is very important! Your protein regimen will totally work, so you have no reason to stress. Look forward to it, rather than worrying about it. Then when you get there, have an *awesome time*. This convinces your body that there is no emergency, that everything is going great. With stress hormones out of the picture, your body has no reason to stockpile fat. When you're at the party, your body will be having it's very own fat-burning party!

SPLURGE SECRET #2: THE SUGAR BINGE.

Each year, my niece's soccer team has an annual pie-making contest. Naturally, her apple pie is the best. But just to make sure, I have to try all the others. Maybe your sugar-coma–inducing event will be Halloween or Easter, or a Valentine's Day chocolate fest. Maybe it will be birthday cake, or it's a holiday dessert buffet. Whatever it is, you *know* exactly how you're going to act. You're going to eat the sweets. You've got to live it up once in a while, right?

Absolutely. Fortunately, you can prepare your metabolism to handle the occasional onslaught of sweet stuff by doing four things:

1. EAT NATURAL SUGARS ALL DAY. HAVE FRUIT AT BREAKFAST AND FRUIT WITH LUNCH. Whole fruit, no juice. When breakfast and lunch are full of fruit, your body gets nicely and comfortably settled in to an elevated *but stable* blood sugar level. For those two meals, breakfast and lunch, eat like it's Phase 1 for breakfast and Phase 1 for lunch.

2. CHANGE ALL YOUR SNACKS TO PROTEIN-ONLY. This will stabilize your metabolism and prep it to handle any garbage you put in. Eat your snacks like it's Phase 2. Fruit with meals, jerky or slices of meat for snacks.

3. HAVE GOOD FATS FOR DINNER. The fat will slow the rate of sugar delivery. So you'll eat dinner like it is Phase 3 again.

4. ENJOY YOURSELF. Go to the party and whoop it up while you're eating that chocolate truffle torte. Then go dancing. Relish it, and don't you dare feel guilty! Remember: Guilt is more fattening than pork rinds.

SPLURGE SECRET #3: BOOZING IT UP.

If you enjoy a cocktail, a glass of wine, or a frosty mug of beer now and again (like once a week or so), I'm not going to take that pleasure away from you. But there is a way to drink alcohol with the least amount of metabolic damage. You probably already know that your liver has to work hard to process alcohol. True, I'm not being quite so greedy with your liver anymore, now that you've effectively repaired your metabolism, but let's not be too hard on it, either. One drink per week probably won't hurt anything. One drink per day is pushing your liver a little bit hard. Figure out what you're willing to sacrifice, but just remember that alcohol does not *help* your metabolism in any way.

You need your liver to function at its prime, after all. So when you do drink alcohol, here are some things to consider:

- **Organic, sulfite-free wine seems to have the least effect on liver function.** If you are a wine connoisseur, you might want to explore your organic options.

- **If you really want a cocktail, go for the top-shelf liquors**. They are cleaner, with fewer chemicals and fake ingredients for the liver to process. Clear liquors without additives and food colorings are purer, better choices than the cheap stuff. Avoid anything you used to get drunk on in college, or those neon-colored energy drinks that mix caffeine with your alcohol. Otherwise, your waistline will begin to resemble a pony keg rather than a six-pack. **Always drink 8 ounces of water for every drink,** in *addition* to your requisite half-your-body-weight ounces. Alcohol is very dehydrating, and this will help your body compensate.

- **Don't drink alcohol alone.** By this I don't mean you can't enjoy a glass of wine at home by yourself after a long day. What I mean is, always balance alcohol with a fairly heavy protein, preferably an animal protein like chicken, turkey, beef, shrimp, or fish (cheese on the nachos doesn't count!).

- **Please do *not* have alcohol in the morning.** Look, I *know* a Bloody Mary at brunch can be tempting, but it will taste just as good without the alcohol. It may always be 5:00 P.M. somewhere, but wait until it is 5:00 P.M. where *you* are.

FAST METABOLISM 911

I have to take a hard stance and act as a guardrail for my clients and my readers. If you start taking the turns too fast and begin to veer off the road I want to be here with my stern rules to keep you from going over the proverbial cliff and falling off this diet. If you break my hard-and-fast rules and the guardrail fails you, we must have a way to call 911 and get you the help you need and the healing your wounded metabolism requires. But remember, 911 is for emergencies only, not a way to cheat yourself through a traffic jam!

EMERGENCY #1: I AM STUCK AND CAN'T FIND ANYTHING PHASE-SPECIFIC TO EAT

Try to get your hands on some protein. It is the least likely to be stored as fat and the most likely to preserve the muscle from being cannibalized. Plus it's easy to find; even gas stations carry hard boiled eggs or cans of tuna. Then get right back into your phase-specific rhythm.

EMERGENCY #2: I LEFT THE HOUSE AND SKIPPED BREAKFAST

Don't stress! That will only make things worse from a hormonal perspective. We do not want to signal the adrenals to ramp up cortisol production. Take deep breaths to lower cortisol output, then get food ASAP. Stick to your phase-specific snack or meal, but to make up for the lost time, make sure it includes a vegetable. This will help keep the body alkalinized and out of stress-based acidosis. For the remainder of the day, stick to your regular schedule and that night, prepare and set out your breakfast for the next morning to prevent it from happening again.

EMERGENCY #3: I CAN'T FIND THE TIME TO MAKE MY WORKOUTS OR I AM INJURED AND CAN'T EXERCISE

You can start a fire without kindling and you can have success on this diet without working out. In Phase 1, doing anything that elevates your heart rate for just a 10- to 20-minute period will make a huge difference. In Phase 2 you get the hormonal benefit of weight lifting even if you only work one muscle. So if you broke your left arm, use your right arm. Doing bicep curls with one arm counts. In Phase 3, deep breathe while you lay in bed at night as you are tying to go to sleep. It will help you sleep better *and* balance out hormones.

EMERGENCY #4: A DRINK FELL IN MY MOUTH AND IN THE SHOCK OF IT ALL I SWALLOWED IT . . . TWICE!

Repent by drinking an additional 8 ounces of water for each alcoholic indiscretion and the next day focus on potassium-rich foods such as cucumbers, basil, parsley, and cilantro. These are natural diuretics and can help rebalance the liver quickly.

EMERGENCY #5: I JUST WASN'T HUNGRY SO I SKIPPED MY SNACK

Oh, you ate. You just ate your own muscle rather than your snack. Remember when you have been in a weight-gaining trend or weight loss has been difficult your hunger signals are likely to be off. Do not wait to get hungry. Eat every 3 to 4 hours. If you have gone longer than that and you suddenly find yourself "starving" be very careful about portions. Do not overeat. Instead, finish your snack or meal and add another snack one hour later. This will stretch out the food delivery to the bloodstream and reduce your risk for fat storage.

EMERGENCY #6: I STARTED THE DIET AND HAD TO STOP BEFORE FINISHING THE 28 DAYS—CAN I GIVE IT ANOTHER TRY?

Yes. This diet will always be here for you, and healthy, metabolism-enhancing eating at any time can promote healing and health in your body. Believe me, I understand that life happens. I had a client that was with me for three years and didn't lose a single pound. The mochas, sudden business trips, divorce, deaths in her family, caring for an elderly parent and just life were enough to pull her off the program again and again. I was impressed we were able to keep her from gaining and keep her diabetes in line. Then one day the stars aligned and she did four straight months of the Fast Metabolism Diet. She lost 65 pounds. I am patient and ready when you are! I've got a full 28 days to give you.

These are my survival strategies when real life happens and gets in the way of our "perfect" health plan. I know I said that you were mine for only 28 days, but I want you to know the door is always open and the same principles of healing and repair of the metabolism can be applied to the healing and repair of arthritis, high cholesterol, diabetes, and fatigue.

In my practice I still have clients that I saw the first week I opened my doors. I have watched my clients' families grow and expand. I've celebrated their successes with them and shared in their heartaches and hardships.

Some, I haven't seen in a long time. I got a referral recently from a past client whom I hadn't seen in three years—not since he had come in and successfully lost 40 pounds with me. The friend he referred to me went on and on about his friend, my original client, and how great he looked, and what a killer body he had. It was so great to hear how he was still thriving.

I wasn't surprised. That's how the Fast Metabolism Diet works. You learn it, you live it, you love it, and you never go back. He had learned how to live and eat to maintain and nurture his metabolism for life. Food is the most worthy of medicines, so keep the momentum of the last few weeks and go out and live!

But remember that I'm here for you. I am your nutritionist for life, and through the website, my clinics, and any forthcoming books, I will continue to provide you with new, innovative, and easy ways to get healthy, stay healthy, and embrace life. I want you to be singing the praises of the Fast Metabolism Diet for years to come because it finally got you out of the vicious cycle of dieting. Now you will be living the Fast Metabolism lifestyle, enjoying delicious recipes from the cookbook, interacting with a community dedicated to health and wellness, and having the resources that you need to maintain your killer new body!

And if you have reached your goal weight and you're totally comfortable and happy at the weight you've achieved, please, right now, go out and have your clothes tailored or buy a new pair of jeans. Because we are never going back there again!

Finally, before we meet again, this is what I have in mind for your future:

I want you to have a long life full of health and love.

I want you to count your treasures and not your calories.

I want you to have energy to experience joy.

I want you to have the resources to repair your body whenever necessary.

I want you to love food and all that it can do for you.

Above all, I want you to go out and flaunt your fast metabolism for the world to see and fully indulge in the pleasure of the Fast Metabolism lifestyle.

CHAPTER ELEVEN

HAYLIE
POMROY

Four Weeks' Worth of Recipes

I hope I've seduced you into a new love for cooking, if you didn't already love it, because home-cooked real food is by far the best way to eat to maintain a fast metabolism. But you need recipes, and I've got great ones! Each recipe in this chapter is marked according to the phase for which it is appropriate, and they are all delicious. Many of them have become favorites for my family and also for many of my clients. I know you'll enjoy them, too.

PHASE 1 RECIPES

Don't be caught hungry without a Crash Stash snack! During Phase 1, snack time is all about fruit, so keep travel-worthy fruit stashed in your desk, in your car, in your purse. Apples, oranges, and tangerines travel well.

One of my favorite fruits is mango, but fresh mangos aren't really practical for eating at my desk. When I peel and eat a mango and chew on the seed, I make a big mess! But I figured out a way to have mangos on the run. I just stash a bag of frozen mangos in my purse or car. By mid-morning snack time, they are defrosted but still chilled and absolutely delicious! Buy a large bag of frozen mangos and divide it up into individual baggies so you can have mangos whenever you want them.

PHASE 1 BREAKFASTS

Frozen Mango Fat-Burning Smoothie

Oatmeal Fruit Smoothie

Oatmeal

Strawberry French Toast

PHASE 1 SALADS, SANDWICHES, SOUPS, AND CHILIS

Tuna, Green Apple, and Spinach Salad

Open-Faced Chicken/Turkey Sandwich

Sprouted-Grain Turkey Wrap

Chicken and Barley Soup

Turkey or Buffalo Chili

Turkey, White Bean, and Kale Soup

Phase 1 Salad Dressing and Veggie Dip

Chicken and Broccoli Bowl

Chicken Sausage with Brown Rice Fusilli

Italian Chicken and Wild Rice

Filet Mignon with Brown Rice

Pork Tenderloin with Broccoli

PHASE 1 SNACKS

Baked Cinnamon Grapefruit

Cacao Asian Pear

Fat-Burning Watermelon Slices

Watermelon Smoothie

FROZEN MANGO FAT-BURNING SMOOTHIE

PHASE 1

Serves 1

1 cup frozen mango (or strawberries or pineapple)
½ cup ice cubes
½ lemon
¼ teaspoon Stevia or Xylitol (optional)
2 mint leaves or ¼ teaspoon peppermint tea leaves

Add the mango and ice to a blender along with ¾ cup water. Juice the lemon and add along with the Stevia or Xylitol. Sprinkle the mint into the mix and puree until smooth. Enjoy with 8 to 10 rice crackers.

OATMEAL FRUIT SMOOTHIE

PHASE 1

Serves 1

1 cup steel-cut oats, cooked
1 cup frozen fruit, such as pineapple or strawberries
½ cup ice cubes
1 packet Stevia or Xylitol
Ground cinnamon, to taste

Put the oats in a blender and pulse until they reach a powdery consistency. Turn off the blender and add ½ cup water. Incorporate the remaining ingredients into the mix and blend until smooth. Serve.

OATMEAL

PHASE 1

Serves 2

I like to make the whole box of oats at one sitting and then freeze it with berries, cinnamon, and Stevia in 2 cup serving portions. This way, I can easily remove them from the freezer and reheat in minutes when doing Phase 1 again. You can also cook steel-cut oats overnight in a slow cooker.

1 cup steel-cut oats
2 cups fresh berries
Stevia and ground cinnamon, to taste

Add the oats to 4 cups water in a large bowl. Cover and put in fridge to soak overnight. The next morning, place the mixture in a saucepan and simmer for approximately 30 minutes. Stir constantly to keep from sticking. When the oats finish cooking, top with the berries, then sprinkle with Stevia and cinnamon.

STRAWBERRY FRENCH TOAST

PHASE 1

Serves 1

1 egg white
1 teaspoon vanilla extract
¼ teaspoon ground cinnamon
1 slice sprouted-grain bread
1 cup frozen strawberries
2 teaspoons lemon juice
$^1/_8$ teaspoon Stevia or Xylitol

Whisk together the egg white, vanilla, and cinnamon in a small mixing bowl. Soak the bread well in the mix, coating both sides.

Heat a nonstick skillet and place the bread onto the hot surface, turning occasionally to toast both sides.

While it cooks, heat the strawberries in a pan over low heat. When they are halfway softened, add the lemon juice and Stevia or Xylitol and cook until warm. Immediately pour over the French toast and eat!

TUNA, GREEN APPLE, AND SPINACH SALAD

PHASE 1

Serves 1

5-ounce can solid white tuna, packed in water
1 cup chopped green apple (or red apple or pineapple)
½ cup peeled and diced cucumber
½ cup diced carrot
1 tablespoon minced red onion
½ lemon
1 to 2 cups fresh spinach

Drain the tuna well and put in a small mixing bowl. Add the apple, cucumber, carrot, and red onion and mix well.

Juice the lemon into the mixture and stir well. Serve over the spinach.

Note: If preferred, use balsamic vinegar to taste instead of lemon, but no oil.

OPEN-FACED TURKEY SANDWICH

PHASE 1

Serves 1

1 slice sprouted-grain bread
1 tablespoon prepared mustard
2 large lettuce leaves
2 slices nitrate-free turkey or chicken deli meat
A few slices red onion
Several tomato slices
Sea salt and freshly ground pepper

Spread the bread with the mustard. Layer the lettuce leaves and turkey slices on top. Add the onion and tomato. Season with salt and pepper. Serve.

SPROUTED-GRAIN TURKEY WRAP

PHASE 1

Serves 1

4 strips turkey bacon or ½ cup lean ground turkey (about 4 ounces)
¼ teaspoon sea salt
¼ teaspoon dry mustard
¼ teaspoon black pepper
¼ teaspoon dried oregano
1 to 2 tablespoons prepared mustard
1 sprouted-grain tortilla

½ to 1 cup dark leafy greens, such as arugula or spring mix or spinach

½ ripe medium tomato, sliced

Cook the turkey bacon or ground turkey in a nonstick pan. Season with the sea salt, dry mustard, pepper, and oregano.

Spread the prepared mustard on the tortilla, and add the greens and tomato sliced.

Top with the bacon or ground turkey, roll tortilla up, and enjoy!

CHICKEN AND BARLEY SOUP

PHASE 1

Serves 10 (portion size: 3 cups)

4 cups chicken broth

4 cups vegetable broth

2½ pounds skinless, boneless chicken breast, cubed

1 cup diced onion

1 tablespoon crushed garlic

1 whole bay leaf

¼ teaspoon sea salt

¼ teaspoon black pepper

2 cups peeled and cubed butternut squash

2 cups cubed yellow summer squash

2 cups cubed zucchini

1 cup broccoli florets

1 cup chopped fresh mushrooms

2 cups barley

Put 4 cups of water into a large soup pot and add the broths. Add the chicken, onion, garlic, bay leaf, salt, and pepper. Bring all ingredients to a boil. Turn down the heat to low and allow the soup to simmer for 1 hour.

Add the vegetables and barley to the soup pot. Bring back to a boil and simmer on low for another hour or two, until vegetables are desired texture.

TURKEY OR BUFFALO CHILI

Serves approximately 8 (single portion: 1½ cups)

Please note: Because this recipe contains such a large amount of starchy legumes, it counts as a Grain as well as Protein and Veggie servings. No need to add an additional Grain to the meal, even if the meal map specifies a Grain.

1 to 1½ pounds lean ground turkey or buffalo meat
½ cup diced red onion, or more, if desired
2 tablespoons parsley or cilantro
1 heaping tablespoon chili powder
1 tablespoon minced garlic
½ teaspoon crushed red pepper flakes (see Note)
15-ounce can white beans
15-ounce can kidney beans
15-ounce can black beans
15-ounce can pinto beans
15-ounce can lentils or adzuki beans
4 cups chopped zucchini
4 cups (32 ounces) organic bell pepper–tomato soup or plain tomato soup
   (Just be sure it is not milk-based. For brands I use, visit my website.)
1 heaping teaspoon sea salt

Brown the turkey in a skillet and drain.

Turn a slow cooker to high setting. Add the meat, onion, parsley, chili powder, garlic, and red pepper flakes to the pot. Stir, cover, and set aside.

Open and partially drain all five cans of beans; I leave a little liquid in to make my chili a little juicier. Add the beans, zucchini, and soup to the cooker. Stir well. Keep the cooker set on high for 4 to 5 hours, or adjust heat to low and simmer for 6 to 8 hours.

Stir and taste occasionally, adjusting seasonings as needed. Add the salt just before serving to best preserve its nutrients.

Note: Adds a little kick, and you can always add more when serving if you like it with kick, but the rest of the family doesn't. Also, I will make this chili before I get the kids up in the morning and set it to low so it is hot and ready to go for dinner. Or, if I am slow cooking for the future, I will throw it in right before I go to bed and fridge or freeze it in the morning before I leave for work.

TURKEY, WHITE BEAN, AND KALE SOUP

PHASE 1

Serves 8

2 pounds lean ground turkey
3 cups diced red onions
2 cups diced celery (including green tops)
2 tablespoons minced garlic
1 tablespoon minced ginger
8 cups vegetable broth
6 cups peeled and cubed kabocha or butternut squash
6 cups roughly chopped kale (ribs removed)
15-ounce can baby butter beans, drained and rinsed
15-ounce can great northern beans, drained and rinsed
15-ounce can adzuki or black beans, drained and rinsed
2 teaspoons dried basil
2 teaspoons dried thyme
1 teaspoon ground cumin
½ teaspoon sea salt
¼ teaspoon freshly ground black pepper

In a very large nonstick soup pot, sauté the turkey, onions, celery, garlic, and ginger in 2 tablespoons of water until soft. Add the broth, squash, kale, beans, and spices. Bring to a boil.

Cover the pot, reduce the heat to low, and simmer for 15 to 20 minutes or until the vegetables are tender. Taste and adjust seasonings with salt and pepper as needed.

SALAD DRESSING AND VEGGIE DIP

PHASE 1

Makes about ¾ cup

½ cup fresh or thawed mango chunks

2 teaspoons balsamic vinegar

2 teaspoons chopped fresh cilantro or parsley

1 teaspoon lime juice

¼ teaspoon Stevia or Xylitol

Blend all the ingredients in a blender. Enjoy with cut vegetables!

CHICKEN AND BROCCOLI BOWL

PHASE 1

Serves 4

4 cups vegetable or chicken broth

½ cup chopped red onion

½ cup chopped carrot

½ cup chopped celery

1 tablespoon parsley or cilantro

1 teaspoon minced garlic

2 cups brown rice

1 pound skinless, boneless chicken breast, chopped into 2-inch pieces

4 cups broccoli florets

1 tablespoon lime juice

½ teaspoon minced parsley

½ teaspoon sea salt

½ teaspoon black pepper

Preheat the oven to 375 degrees.

Mix the broth, vegetables (except the broccoli), 1 tablespoon parsley, and garlic in a large pot. Add 1 cup of water and bring to a boil. Add the rice and bring back to a boil. Cover and simmer for 25 minutes. Remove the lid and simmer for 5 more minutes. Set aside.

While the rice cooks, put the chicken and broccoli in a mixing bowl. Add the lime juice, parsley, salt, and pepper. Mix well until the chicken and broccoli are coated with the flavorings. Transfer the chicken and broccoli mixture to a larger baking pan, spreading it evenly in the bottom with a spatula. Bake for 30 to 35 minutes.

Remove the chicken from the oven and allow to cool. Divide the rice into four servings. Divide the chicken and broccoli mixture into four equal portions and place on top of the rice. Serve and enjoy. (Don't hesitate to double this recipe and freeze more portions.)

CHICKEN SAUSAGE WITH BROWN RICE FUSILLI

PHASE 1

Serves 4

2 cups brown rice fusilli
16 ounces chicken sausage
2 cups cubed zucchini
1 cup broccoli florets
¼ cup minced red onion
1 tablespoon crushed garlic
¼ teaspoon sea salt
⅛ teaspoon black pepper

Prepare the pasta according to package directions, being careful to not overcook the pasta. When the pasta is done, strain and rinse it. Set aside.

Cut the chicken sausage into 1-inch pieces.

Preheat a large nonstick skillet. Add 1 tablespoon of water and stir in the sausage, onion, and garlic. Cook on medium heat until lightly browned. Incorporate the zucchini, broccoli, salt, and pepper, and cook until vegetables are crisp-tender, about 3–5 minutes.

Add the pasta to the skillet and toss until warmed through. Serve immediately.

ITALIAN CHICKEN AND WILD RICE

PHASE 1

Serves 6–8 (portion size: 1½ to 2 cups)

2½ pounds skinless, boneless chicken breast, cubed
2 cups chicken broth
1 cup wild rice, rinsed and drained
¼ cup diced onion
½ teaspoon minced garlic
2 cups chopped fresh mushrooms
14.5-ounce can diced tomatoes
1 teaspoon sea salt
½ teaspoon dried oregano
½ teaspoon dried basil
¼ teaspoon freshly ground black pepper

Put the chicken breast, broth, wild rice, onion, and garlic in a slow cooker. Stir in the mushrooms, tomatoes, salt, oregano, basil, and pepper. Cover and simmer for 4 hours on high or 6 hours on low. Serve and enjoy!

FILET MIGNON WITH BROWN RICE

PHASE 1

Serves 4

BROWN RICE

4 cups chicken or vegetable broth
2 cups uncooked brown rice
1 cup diced zucchini
½ cup diced ripe tomatoes

2 tablespoons diced red onion
1 teaspoon (fresh or dried) cilantro
1 teaspoon crushed garlic

FILET MIGNON

Juice of ¼ lemon or lime
½ sprig fresh rosemary
1 teaspoon crushed garlic
$1/8$ teaspoon sea salt
$1/8$ teaspoon black pepper
16-ounce beef filet

Make the rice. Put the broth in a saucepan and bring to a boil. Once boiling, add all the remaining rice ingredients, cover, and bring back to a boil. Allow to simmer, covered, stirring occasionally, for 30 minutes or until desired consistency.

Make the filet. Preheat the broiler with broiler pan in place. Mix the lemon or lime juice, rosemary, garlic, sea salt, and black pepper and rub generously all over the filet. Broil the filet on high until desired doneness. Serve with the rice.

PORK TENDERLOIN WITH BROCCOLI

PHASE 1

Serves 1

Juice of ½ lemon
¼ teaspoon minced garlic
¼ teaspoon dried parsley
$1/8$ teaspoon dried rosemary
$1/8$ teaspoon dried oregano
$1/8$ teaspoon sea salt
Pinch of Stevia
Pinch of ground cinnamon

4 to 6 ounces sliced pork tenderloin
3 cups broccoli florets

Prepare the marinade: Mix the lemon juice, garlic, parsley, rosemary, oregano, salt, Stevia, and cinnamon in a small bowl. Put the pork in a large zippered plastic bag and pour the marinade into the bag. Close tightly. Marinate in the refrigerator for a minimum of 30 minutes, although over-night is best.

Prepare a charcoal or gas grill. Drain and grill the pork over high heat, turning only one to two times, about 5 to 6 minutes total. (A high tem-perature keeps the tenderloin from drying out.)

Remove the tenderloin from the grill and keep warm. Place the broccoli florets in a grill basket and onto the grill and cook for 30 seconds on each side, to char. Remove and serve with the tenderloin.

Note: If you don't have a grill, you can broil the tenderloin. Heat the broiler pan first, then add the loin, and serve over a cup of brown rice.

BAKED CINNAMON GRAPEFRUIT
PHASE 1
Serves 1

1 pink grapefruit
¼ teaspoon of cinnamon
Pinch of cardamom (optional)
Pinch of nutmeg (optional)

Peel and section grapefruit. Sprinkle with cinnamon, cardamom, and nutmeg. Bake for 20 minutes at 375 degrees or until cinnamon has cara-melized.

CACAO ASIAN PEAR

PHASE 1

Serves 1

1 Asian pear
½ to 1 teaspoon cacao powder

Slice pear and sprinkle with cacao powder. Eat raw or bake for 10 minutes (or microwave for 30 seconds) before serving.

FAT-BURNING WATERMELON SLICES

PHASE 1

Serves 1

1 cup sliced watermelon
¼ teaspoon chili powder
1 teaspoon lime juice

Sprinkle the watermelon with chili powder and then pour lime juice on top.

WATERMELON SMOOTHIE

PHASE 1

Serves 1

1 cup watermelon cubes
2 tablespoons lime juice
2 drops peppermint extract
1 mint leaf

Freeze watermelon. Blend watermelon cubes in blender with lime juice and peppermint extract and 1 cup ice. Garnish with mint leaf.

I often recommend organic foods and unprocessed foods, but remember that because they aren't filled with chemical preservatives, they don't last as long. So when you cook something fresh, cook multiple servings and keep what you don't eat in the freezer, in individual serving containers, marked according to phase. The freezer will become your best friend on this plan, especially if you are busy and only have time to cook once or twice a week. Naturally preserved meats and sprouted-grain breads, in particular, should be kept frozen until the day before you're ready to eat them to prevent spoilage, molding, and fermentation.

PHASE 2

PHASE 2 CRASH STASH

During Phase 2, snack time is all about lean meat, and my favorite easy Crash Stash form is jerky. However, a lot of jerky can be filled with preservatives like nitrates. While some places have nitrate-free jerky (but look out for sugar in the ingredient list; I like the Shelton's brand), it's also really easy to make your own. I had a client who loved jerky, so she made enough at one time for all eight days and sixteen snacks she needed for Phase 2 days. She helped me write the homemade jerky recipe for this book, which you can find on page 212.

My friend's only challenge was keeping her family away from that scrumptious homemade jerky. Finally, I told her to portion it out in freezer bags, then put them in a brown paper bag in the freezer labeled "Yucky Phase 2 Snacks." It worked! She got away with it, and now her family can't believe how much weight she's lost. You can do what she did, right down to the family fake-out. It's totally worth it to have homemade jerky available for every Phase 2 snack.

Many of my clients love to wrap slices of nitrate-free deli meat around a few celery sticks, asparagus spears, or any other portable Phase 2 veggie. You can simply buy a package of sliced roast beef or turkey, divide it into ziplock bags (about 3 to 4 thin slices per bag) with some veggies, then stash the bags in the refrigerator for easy, ready-made snack packs.

PHASE 2 BREAKFASTS

Spanish Egg White Scramble

Egg White, Mushroom, and Spinach Omelet

Turkey Bacon with Celery, Sea Salt, and Lime

PHASE 2 SALADS, SANDWICHES, AND SOUPS

Tuna Salad–Stuffed Red Pepper

Tuna and Cucumber Salad

Steak and Spinach Salad

Roast Beef, Horseradish, and Cucumber Wrap

Roast Beef, Mustard, and Lettuce Wrap

Steak and Asparagus Lettuce Wrap

Sliced Chicken Wrap

Chicken and Veggie Soup

Beef, Kale, and Leek Soup

Southwestern Beef and Cabbage Soup

Phase 2 Salad Dressing and Veggie Dip

PHASE 2 MAIN COURSES

Spicy Red Pepper Fish with Lemon-Garlic Kale

Broiled Halibut with Broccoli

Baked Cinnamon-Mustard Chicken and Lemon-Garlic Spinach

New York Strip Steak with Steamed Broccoli

Stuffed Red Bell Pepper

Pepperoncini Pork Roast

PHASE 2 SNACKS

Turkey Jerky

Smoked Salmon and Cucumbers

Oysters Canapé

Roast Beef-Stuffed Green Chile Pepper

Oysters on the Half Shell

Stuffed Mushrooms

SPANISH EGG WHITE SCRAMBLE

PHASE 2

Serves 1

1 tablespoon chopped onion
1 tablespoon chopped shallot
1 tablespoon minced garlic
1 tablespoon minced green chile pepper
½ cup chopped fresh spinach
3 egg whites (or ½ cup egg whites)
¼ teaspoon dried or 1 teaspoon fresh cilantro or parsley
¼ teaspoon crushed red pepper flakes
Pinch of sea salt

In a nonstick pan, heat a teaspoon of water and cook the onion, shallot, garlic, and chile until soft. Stir in the spinach until wilted. Mix in the egg whites and scramble. Allow the eggs to cook until desired consistency. Sprinkle with parsley, red pepper flakes, and salt before serving.

EGG WHITE, MUSHROOM, AND SPINACH OMELET
PHASE 2
Serves 1

1 tablespoon chopped onion
1 tablespoon chopped shallot
1 tablespoon minced garlic
½ cup chopped fresh spinach
¹/₃ cup chopped fresh mushrooms
3 egg whites (or ½ cup egg whites)
Pinch of sea salt

Heat the onion, shallot, and garlic in a nonstick skillet until soft. Stir in the spinach and mushrooms, cooking until the spinach wilts. Mix in the egg whites. Allow the eggs to cook until desired consistency. Sprinkle with sea salt before serving.

TURKEY BACON WITH CELERY, SEA SALT, AND LIME
PHASE 2
Serves 1

4 slices nitrate-free turkey bacon (approximately 3 to 4 ounces)
2 long celery stalks
1 teaspoon lime juice
Sea salt to taste

Cook the turkey bacon in a nonstick pan or skillet for 4 minutes on one side and 3 minutes on the other. Season the celery stalks with lime juice and salt. Serve together.

TUNA SALAD–STUFFED RED PEPPER

PHASE 2

Serves 1

5-ounce can tuna, packed in water
3 small Persian cucumbers, finely chopped
½ cup fresh basil, cut in chiffonade
2 tablespoons finely chopped red onion
2 tablespoons lemon juice
1 tablespoon prepared mustard
Pinch of sea salt
Pinch of black pepper
1 red bell pepper, washed, halved, and cored

Drain the tuna. Put into a small mixing bowl and add the cucumbers, basil, and onion. Stir well. Fold in the lemon juice, mustard, salt, and pepper. Spoon the tuna mixture into the red pepper halves. Serve and enjoy!

TUNA AND CUCUMBER SALAD

PHASE 2

Serves 1

5-ounce can tuna, packed in water
3 small Persian cucumbers, chopped
½ cup basil, cut in chiffonade
2 tablespoons minced red onion
2 tablespoons lemon juice
1 tablespoon prepared mustard
Pinch of sea salt
Pinch of black pepper
2 cups chopped fresh spinach, cabbage, or kale
2–4 tablespoons Phase 2 Salad Dressing (page 207)

Drain the tuna well and put in a small mixing bowl. Stir in the cucumbers, basil, onion, lemon juice, and mustard. Add salt and pepper to taste. Serve the tuna salad over a bed of spinach, cabbage, or kale. Drizzle with dressing.

STEAK AND SPINACH SALAD

PHASE 2

Serves 1

4 to 5 ounces New York strip steak
½ teaspoon minced garlic
½ teaspoon sea salt
⅛ teaspoon pepper
2 cups chopped fresh spinach
½ cup chopped cucumber
¼ cup chopped red onion
¼ cup chopped red or green chile pepper
¼ cup chopped red bell pepper
½ lime, squeezed
1 to 2 tablespoons fresh cilantro
2 to 4 tablespoons Phase 2 Salad Dressing (page 207)

Preheat the broiler, and put the broiler pan in to get hot. Trim excess fat off the steak. Rub both sides of the steak with the garlic, salt, and pepper.

Place the meat in the hot broiler pan and broil to desired doneness, 5 to 7 minutes (you can butterfly or slice the steak in half if you want it well done without charring the outside).

While the steak broils, toss the spinach, cucumber, onion, chile, and bell pepper together in a large salad bowl. Top the mixture with the lime juice and cilantro. Set aside.

Slice the steak into 1½-inch strips and serve on top of the salad and veggie mix. Drizzle with dressing before serving.

ROAST BEEF, HORSERADISH, AND CUCUMBER WRAP

PHASE 2

Serves 1

1 to 2 tablespoons prepared horseradish
2 to 3 ounces nitrate-free deli roast beef slices
1 cucumber, peeled and cut into spears
Sea salt, to taste

Spread the horseradish on the roast beef slices and wrap around the cucumber spears. Add salt. Serve and enjoy.

ROAST BEEF, MUSTARD, AND LETTUCE WRAP

PHASE 2

Serves 1

2 to 3 ounces nitrate-free deli roast beef slices
1 to 2 tablespoons prepared mustard
2 to 4 large romaine leaves
Cilantro (optional)
Crushed red pepper flakes (optional)
Lime juice (optional)

Spread the mustard on top of the roast beef slices. Then wrap with the romaine leaves. Sprinkle with cilantro, red pepper flakes, or lime juice and serve.

STEAK AND ASPARAGUS LETTUCE WRAPS

PHASE 2

Serves 2

An 8-ounce beefsteak, cut into strips
8 asparagus spears, trimmed

½ lime, juiced

½ teaspoon minced garlic

½ teaspoon dried or 1 teaspoon fresh cilantro

½ teaspoon sea salt

¼ teaspoon black pepper

¼ teaspoon crushed red pepper flakes

Mustard or balsamic vinegar to taste

4 large romaine leaves

Preheat the broiler and put the broiler pan in the oven.

Make a foil pouch for the steak and asparagus. Whisk together the lime juice, garlic, cilantro, salt, pepper, and red pepper flakes in a small bowl. Drizzle onto the steak and asparagus. Seal the pouch. Put the foil pouch on the broiler pan and broil for 20 to 25 minutes, depending on how well done you like your steak.

Remove the pouch from the oven and carefully open, allowing the heat to escape and the meat to cool.

Pour the pouch liquid into a small bowl and toss with a little mustard or balsamic vinegar.

On a serving plate, arrange 2 romaine leaves. Spoon half the steak and asparagus mixture onto each leaf and drizzle sauce over the top. Place the remaining 2 leaves on top, roll up, and enjoy!

Note: If you have leftovers or want to double the recipe, set aside the rest of the steak and asparagus for tomorrow's lunch, wrap in lettuce leaves, and drizzle with Phase 2 Salad Dressing (page 207), if desired.

SLICED CHICKEN WRAP

PHASE 2

Serves 1

1 to 2 tablespoons prepared mustard
2 to 3 ounces nitrate-free deli sliced chicken (or turkey)
2 to 3 romaine lettuce leaves
Fresh cilantro (optional)
Crushed red pepper flakes (optional)
Lime juice (optional)

Spread the mustard on the chicken and wrap in the romaine leaves. Sprinkle with cilantro, red pepper flakes, or lime juice before serving.

CHICKEN AND VEGGIE SOUP

PHASE 2

Serves 6 to 8 (single portion: 3 cups)

2 pounds chicken breast, skin removed
1 cup chopped onion
6 to 8 garlic cloves, minced
8 cups chicken broth
8 cups chopped fresh or frozen vegetables, including cabbage, broccoli,
    celery, spinach, kale, asparagus, leeks, chives, and mushrooms
1 tablespoon parsley or cilantro
1 teaspoon fresh or dried rosemary
½ teaspoon fresh or dried basil
½ teaspoon fresh or dried oregano
¼ teaspoon fresh or dried thyme
1 bay leaf
Sea salt and white and black pepper

Put the chicken in a large soup pot along with the broth and 8 cups of water. Add the vegetables and herbs. Bring to a boil, then lower the heat and simmer for 1 hour.

Let cool, then remove the chicken and debone. Add chicken meat to the soup, reheat, season with salt and pepper, and serve.

BEEF, KALE, AND LEEK SOUP

PHASE 2

Serves 6 to 8

2 pounds boneless stew beef or lamb (or substitute)
4 cups (32 ounces) vegetable broth
4 cups (32 ounces) beef broth
3 cups chopped kale (ribs removed)
2 cups baby spinach
2 cups sliced fresh mushrooms
1 cup chopped leek, green and white parts
1 cup chopped celery
6 green onions, chopped (green and white parts)
¼ cup chopped red onion
1 tablespoon minced garlic
1 tablespoon sea salt
½ teaspoon ground black pepper

Brown meat, then put all ingredients in a slow cooker and cook on low for 6 to 8 hours or on high for 4 to 5 hours.

SOUTHWESTERN BEEF AND CABBAGE SOUP

PHASE 2

Serves 6 to 8 (portion size: 3 cups)

½ cup chopped red onion
2 tablespoons minced garlic
2 pounds boneless stew beef

8-ounce can fire-roasted green chiles, diced
1 tablespoon minced cilantro
½ teaspoon crushed red pepper flakes
½ teaspoon black pepper
4 cups beef broth
4 cups vegetable broth
8 cups water
12 cups shredded green cabbage
2 tablespoons sea salt

In a very large nonstick pot over medium heat, cook the onion and garlic with 2 tablespoons water until soft. Add the beef, chiles, cilantro, red pepper flakes, and pepper. Stir until the spices coat the beef.

Pour in the broths, plus 8 cups of water. Increase the heat to high. When the soup comes to a boil, reduce to medium. Add the cabbage and salt. Stirring occasionally, simmer for approximately 1 hour. Serve immediately.

Note: You can also throw everything into a 6-quart slow cooker and let it cook on low for 6 to 8 hours.

SALAD DRESSING AND VEGGIE DIP

PHASE 2

Makes about ¾ cup

½ cup chopped peeled cucumber
1 garlic clove
3 teaspoons balsamic or apple cider vinegar
2 teaspoons cilantro or parsley
1 teaspoon dill
½ teaspoon Stevia or Xylitol
¹/₈ teaspoon sea salt

Place all ingredients in a blender and blend until smooth.

SPICY RED PEPPER FISH WITH LEMON-GARLIC KALE

Serves 1

1 tablespoon lime juice
1 teaspoon chili paste
¼ teaspoon crushed red pepper flakes
½ teaspoon chopped cilantro
Pinch of sea salt
Pinch of ground black pepper
6 ounces white fish fillet (halibut, cod, dory, flounder)

LEMON-GARLIC KALE
1 tablespoon lemon juice
1 teaspoon minced garlic
3 cups chopped kale (thick ribs removed)

In a small mixing bowl, combine the lime juice, chili paste, red pepper flakes, cilantro, salt, and pepper. Put the fish into a foil-lined pan and drizzle marinade over it.

Preheat the oven to 350 degrees. Bake fish, uncovered, for 20 to 30 minutes depending on the thickness of the fish.

While fish bakes, combine 1 tablespoon of water in a nonstick pan with the lemon juice and garlic.

Add the kale and cook on medium-low heat until tender but still bright green.

Season with salt and pepper, and serve with the fish.

BROILED HALIBUT WITH BROCCOLI

PHASE 2

Serves 1

1 teaspoon lime or lemon juice
½ teaspoon Stevia or Xylitol
½ teaspoon dry mustard
Pinch of ground cinnamon (optional)
6 ounces halibut or other white fish fillet
2 cups broccoli florets
Sea salt
Freshly ground black pepper

Preheat the broiler with broiler pan in place.

In a small mixing bowl, combine the lime or lemon juice with the Stevia, mustard, and cinnamon. Rub generously into the fish to flavor it. Using an oven mitt, remove the broiler pan, put the fish on the hot pan, and broil for 12 to 15 minutes, or until fish begins to flake.

While the fish broils, steam the broccoli. Bring 1 to 2 inches of water to a boil in either a steaming double pan or with a wire steaming tray. Cover and steam broccoli for 4 to 6 minutes, or until easily pierced with a fork. Season with sea salt and pepper before serving with the fish.

BAKED CINNAMON-MUSTARD CHICKEN AND LEMON-GARLIC SPINACH

PHASE 2

Serves 6 to 8

2 tablespoons lemon juice
¼ teaspoon ground cinnamon
1 teaspoon dry mustard
1 teaspoon Stevia or Xylitol
2 pounds skinless, boneless chicken breast, washed and patted dry

LEMON-GARLIC SPINACH

1 tablespoon lemon juice
1 teaspoon minced garlic
3 cups baby spinach
Sea salt and black pepper

Preheat the oven to 350 degrees. While it warms, prepare the seasoning for the chicken.

Combine the lemon juice, cinnamon, mustard, and sweetener in a small mixing bowl.

Put the chicken in a baking dish. Pour the seasoning over it, cover the dish with foil, and put in the oven. Bake the chicken for 30 minutes.

Turn up the heat to 400 degrees and remove the foil. Bake, uncovered, for an additional 10 minutes.

Prepare the spinach. In a nonstick pan, use 1 tablespoon of water and the lemon juice to cook the garlic and spinach. Season with salt and pepper.

NEW YORK STRIP STEAK WITH STEAMED BROCCOLI

PHASE 2

Serves 1

4-ounce New York strip steak (shell steak)
½ teaspoon minced garlic
½ teaspoon sea salt
1/8 teaspoon black pepper
3 cups broccoli florets

Preheat the broiler with broiler pan in place. Trim excess fat off the steak. Rub both sides with the garlic, salt, and pepper. Put the steak on the hot pan and broil to desired doneness, 5 to 10 minutes. (If you want the steak well done without a charred exterior, butterfly the steak or slice the steak in half.)

While the steak is broiling, steam the broccoli. Bring 1 to 2 inches of water to a boil in either a steaming double pan or with a wire steaming tray. Cover and steam for approximately 4 to 6 minutes, or until easily pierced with a fork.

Season with sea salt and pepper before serving with the steak.

Note: I like to make an additional strip steak to slice and serve on a salad for the next day's lunch or dinner.

STUFFED RED BELL PEPPER

PHASE 2

Serves 6

1½ pounds lean ground beef
1 cup chopped red onion
1 cup diced celery
3 tablespoons chopped cilantro
3 tablespoons minced garlic
1½ teaspoons sea salt
1 teaspoon ground black pepper
1 teaspoon dried oregano
1 teaspoon dried basil
1 cup baby spinach
6 red bell peppers

Preheat the oven to 375 degrees. In a large nonstick skillet over medium heat, lightly brown the beef and onion. Turn the heat to low and add the celery, cilantro, garlic, salt, black pepper, oregano, and basil. When the beef is completely browned, remove the mixture from the heat and stir in the spinach.

Wash each bell pepper and remove tops, cores, and seeds. Stuff each pepper with ½ to ⅔ cup of the beef mixture. Put the peppers in a glass baking dish and pour 2 tablespoons of water into the bottom. Cover with foil and bake for 50 minutes.

Remove the stuffed peppers from the oven and take off the foil. Turn up the oven to 400 degrees and cook for an additional 10 minutes. Allow to cool somewhat before serving.

PEPPERONCINI PORK ROAST

PHASE 2

Serves 8

2 pounds boneless pork roast
1 cup minced pepperoncini
1 cup pepperoncini juice
1 teaspoon black pepper
½ teaspoon sea salt
¼ teaspoon dried oregano
¼ teaspoon dried basil
⅛ teaspoon dried rosemary
⅛ teaspoon dry mustard
4 cups chopped broccoli, spinach, or asparagus, steamed

Put all the ingredients except the vegetable in a slow cooker and simmer on low for 6 to 8 hours or on high for 4 to 5 hours. Serve with the steamed broccoli, spinach, or asparagus.

TURKEY JERKY

PHASE 2

Makes 4 to 6 servings

This jerky can also be made with organic beef round steak, buffalo, halibut, or other meat.

1 to 1½ pounds organic turkey breast steaks
¼ cup tamari

Juice of 1 lemon or lime
½ teaspoon onion salt
¼ teaspoon garlic powder
¼ teaspoon black pepper
$^1/_8$ teaspoon sea salt
$^1/_8$ teaspoon crushed red pepper flakes

Trim and discard all fat from the meat. Cut into strips approximately 5 inches long and ½ inch wide. In a large, resealable plastic bag, combine the remaining ingredients. Add the meat to the bag, seal bag, and toss to coat. Refrigerate and let marinate for 8 hours or overnight.

Drain and discard the marinade. Put the meat in a dehydrator or in the oven on wire racks with a foil-lined baking sheet underneath. Arrange meat strips ¼ inch apart on racks. Bake uncovered at 200 degrees for 6 to 7 hours, or until meat is dry and leathery.

Remove from the oven; cool completely. Refrigerate or freeze in an airtight container.

SMOKED SALMON AND CUCUMBERS

PHASE 2

Serves 1

3 ounces nitrate-free smoked salmon (with no added sugar)
1 to 2 cups sliced cucumbers
1 teaspoon lime juice
$^1/_8$ teaspoon dill
Pinch of white pepper

Cut the smoked salmon into thin slices if not already sliced. Drizzle the cucumbers with the lime juice and top with the dill and a sprinkle of white pepper. Serve together.

OYSTERS CANAPÉ

PHASE 2

Serves 2

1 large cucumber
1 3-ounce can oysters packed in water
1 teaspoon lemon juice
Sea salt and pepper to taste

Slice the cucumber into ½ inch slices.

Drain oysters.

Top cucumber slices with oysters and squeeze lemon juice on top. Sprinkle with sea salt and pepper.

ROAST BEEF-STUFFED GREEN CHILE PEPPER

PHASE 2

Serves 1

2 ounces nitrate-free roast beef
1 whole Hatch green chile pepper

Cut top off pepper and stuff with roast beef.

OYSTERS ON THE HALF SHELL

PHASE 2

Serves 1

3 raw oysters

Garnish oysters with horseradish and lemon.

STUFFED MUSHROOMS

PHASE 2

Serves 4

8 ounces lean ground beef
¼ cup minced onion
1 cup minced spinach
1 teaspoon garlic
4 large Portobello mushrooms
Sea salt and pepper to taste
4 tablespoons organic vegetable broth

Brown the first four ingredients in a pan. Divide mixture into four and stuff into the mushrooms. Season with salt and pepper to taste.

Pour 1 tablespoon vegetable broth over each mushroom, cover with aluminum foil and bake at 400 degrees for 15 minutes. Serve hot (or freeze and reheat when ready to eat).

PHASE 3 RECIPES

PHASE 3 CRASH STASH

One of the easiest and yummiest Phase 3 snacks is raw nuts and seeds. They contain both a fat and a protein, and they're perfect for taking along with you wherever you go. One of my clients fills up baggies with all four weeks' worth of snacks at once. She puts a handful of raw almonds, raw cashews, raw pistachios, or raw pumpkin seeds in each of 24 baggies, then puts them in a paper bag labeled "Phase 3 Snacks" and pops them in the fridge. Done!

When appropriate, I also sometimes buy bags of precooked frozen shrimp. I divide them, put 8 to 10 shrimp in each container and add a handful of lemon wedges to each portion, then either freeze or refrigerate (if eating the next day). For the next three days, I've got shrimp cocktail to snack on! Add a few slices of avocado and it's a gourmet-quality snack or a first course for dinner.

PHASE 3 BREAKFASTS

B and B Toast

Cucumber Hummus Toast

Egg and Toast with Tomato and Red Onion

Berry Nutty Oatmeal Smoothie

Berry Nutty Oatmeal

PHASE 3 SALADS, SANDWICHES, AND SOUPS

Endive Tuna Salad

Shrimp Salad

Three-Egg Salad

Olive and Tomato Salad

Phase 3 Salad Dressing and Veggie Dip

Hummus Turkey Roll-Up

Avocado and Turkey Lettuce Wrap

Lentil Stew

PHASE 3 MAIN COURSES

Avocado Quesadillas

Sesame Chicken Stir-Fry

Coconut Curry Chicken

Chicken and Quinoa Risotto

Sesame Chicken and Rice

Baked Salmon and Sweet Potatoes

Avocado Chili

Rosemary Pork Roast with Sweet Potato

Shrimp and Veggie Stir-Fry with Quinoa

Coconut Pecan-Crusted Halibut with Artichoke and Dip

PHASE 3 SNACKS

Almond Butter–Stuffed Celery

Nutty Jicama with Lime

White Bean and Dill Hummus

Creamy Guacamole

Sweet Potato Hummus and Cucumbers

B AND B TOAST

PHASE 3

Serves 1

1 slice sprouted-grain bread
2 tablespoons raw nut or seed butter
1 cup berries
Pinch of cinnamon
Pinch of Stevia or Xylitol (optional)
¼ to ½ cup raw jicama
½ teaspoon lime juice

Toast the bread. Spread the nut or seed butter on the toast and top with ½ cup of the berries. Sprinkle with cinnamon and sweetener. Serve with raw jicama sprinkled with Stevia and lime juice and the remaining ½ cup of berries.

CUCUMBER HUMMUS TOAST

PHASE 3

Serves 1

1 slice sprouted-grain bread
⅓ cup hummus
½ cup thinly sliced cucumber
½ medium tomato, sliced
1 basil leaf (optional)
Pinch of sea salt
Pinch of black pepper

Toast the bread. Spread with the hummus and top with the cucumber and tomato slices.

Place the basil leaf on top and sprinkle with salt and pepper.

EGG AND TOAST WITH TOMATO AND RED ONION

PHASE 3

Serves 1

1 slice sprouted-grain bread
1 large egg
¼ teaspoon olive or grapeseed oil
½ medium tomato, sliced*
¼ red onion, sliced
Sea salt
Black pepper

Toast the bread. Meanwhile, fry the egg in a nonstick skillet with oil. When done, place it on the toast and top with the tomato and onion slices. Add sea salt and pepper to taste.

*In this recipe, tomato counts as your Phase 3 fruit.

BERRY NUTTY OATMEAL SMOOTHIE*

PHASE 3

Serves 1

¼ cup oats, steel-cut or old-fashioned
¼ cup raw sunflower seeds
1 cup frozen blackberries, blueberries, or raspberries
½ cup ice cubes
1 packet Stevia
Ground cinnamon, to taste

Put the oats in a blender and pulse until it becomes a powder. Add the sunflower seeds and continue to blend until finely ground. Turn off the blender and add 1 cup of water and the remaining ingredients. Blend until smooth.

*Don't forget to eat with a serving of Phase 3 veggies.

BERRY NUTTY OATMEAL*

PHASE 3

Serves 1

I like to make the whole box of oats at one sitting and then freeze with the berries, cinnamon, and Stevia in 2 cup portions. This way, I can easily remove them from the freezer and reheat in minutes. Add the nuts or seeds after reheating.

¼ cup steel-cut oats
1 cup fresh berries
¼ cup raw nuts or seeds
Stevia
Ground cinnamon

Add the oats to 1 cup water in a bowl. Cover and soak overnight in the fridge. The next morning, simmer the oats and water in a saucepan for approximately 30 minutes. When the oats finish cooking, top with the berries, nuts, or seeds. Add Stevia and cinnamon to taste.

*Don't forget to eat with a serving of Phase 3 veggies.

ENDIVE TUNA SALAD

PHASE 3

Serves 1

The entire recipe can be used for lunch, or half of the recipe can be used as a snack.

5-ounce can solid white tuna packed in water
¼ cup chopped red onion
¼ cup diced celery
¼ cup diced cucumber
¼ cup diced grapefruit sections
1 tablespoon hummus
Pinch of sea salt
Pinch of ground black pepper
Fresh endive leaves

Drain the tuna and place in a small mixing bowl. Stir in the onion, celery, cucumber, and grapefruit. Add the hummus and stir until well combined. Top with salt and pepper to taste.

Scoop the tuna salad onto fresh endive leaves and serve.

SHRIMP SALAD

Serves 1

You can also serve this on an endive boat or a red bell pepper for lunch, or half of the recipe can be used as a snack.

1 cup cherry tomatoes, diced*
¼ cup finely chopped celery
1 tablespoon finely chopped red onion
2 tablespoons safflower mayonnaise or hummus
1 teaspoon lime juice
½ teaspoon cilantro or parsley
6 ounces cooked shrimp
2 to 4 cups fresh spinach or mixed greens

In a small mixing bowl, combine the tomatoes, celery, and onion. Stir in the mayonnaise, lime juice, and cilantro. Fold in the shrimp.

Serve over spinach or mixed greens.

*In this recipe, tomatoes count as your Phase 3 fruit.

THREE-EGG SALAD

PHASE 3

Serves 1

Half this recipe can also be used as a snack.

3 hard-boiled eggs, peeled and 2 yolks removed
½ tablespoon safflower mayonnaise
¾ tablespoon prepared mustard
2 tablespoons diced black olives
2 tablespoons diced cucumber
½ teaspoon finely chopped red onion (optional)

Pinch of sea salt
2 cups fresh spinach or mixed leafy greens

Chop the egg whites and whole egg. Transfer to a small mixing bowl. Add the mayonnaise and mustard; stir until well incorporated. Add the black olives, cucumber, and onion. Sprinkle with sea salt and stir.

Spoon the egg salad over a bed of spinach to serve.

OLIVE AND TOMATO SALAD

PHASE 3

Serves 1

2 plum or Roma tomatoes, chopped
¼ cup diced mixed olives
¼ cup minced red onion
1 tablespoon olive oil
½ tablespoon balsamic vinegar
5 fresh basil leaves, cut in chiffonade
Sea salt
Black pepper

In a salad bowl, combine the tomatoes, olives, and onion. Toss with the oil and vinegar. Top with the fresh basil, and season to taste with salt and pepper.

SALAD DRESSING AND VEGGIE DIP

PHASE 3

Makes ¼ cup

2 tablespoons sesame oil
2 tablespoons lime juice
1 teaspoon crushed garlic

Sea salt
Black pepper

Mix the ingredients, add salt and pepper to taste. Enjoy as a dressing or dip.

HUMMUS TURKEY ROLL-UP

PHASE 3

Serves 1

2 to 3 slices nitrate-free turkey
2 tablespoons hummus

Spread the hummus directly on the turkey slices, roll them up, and enjoy!

AVOCADO AND TURKEY LETTUCE WRAP

PHASE 3

Serves 1

2 to 4 large romaine lettuce leaves*
2 tablespoons hummus
1 tablespoon salsa of choice
½ cup cooked ground turkey
1 cup arugula
½ avocado, sliced thinly
Sea salt and pepper

Spread the lettuce or warm the tortilla in a dry skillet or in the microwave. Top with the hummus and salsa, spreading evenly. Spoon on the turkey. Top with the arugula and avocado, adding salt and pepper to taste. Wrap and enjoy!

*If eating for dinner, you can swap the lettuce leaves with 1 sprouted-grain tortilla, warmed in a dry skillet or microwave.

LENTIL STEW

Serves 4 (single portion: 1½ cups)

1 tablespoon olive oil
1 small onion, diced
3 garlic cloves, minced
½ cup thinly sliced carrot
Sea salt and black pepper
1 16-ounce can cooked lentils, drained and rinsed, or 2 cups cooked
    lentils
Bragg Liquid Aminos, coconut amino acids, or tamari, to taste
¾ cup chicken or vegetable broth

Over medium heat, warm the oil in a 2-quart saucepan. Add the onion and sauté for 7 minutes, until translucent. Add the garlic and sauté for another minute, until fragrant. Add the carrot, salt, and pepper. Cover and stir occasionally until carrot is tender.

Stir in the lentils and Bragg's; simmer for 5 minutes. Add the broth and simmer for 5 more minutes.

AVOCADO QUESADILLAS

PHASE 3

Serves 1

1 sprouted-grain tortilla
Grapeseed oil
Sea salt to taste
Dried or minced fresh oregano, basil, and rosemary
½ avocado, pitted and peeled
Juice of ¼ lime
¼ teaspoon safflower mayonnaise

Preheat the oven to 350 degrees. Lightly spread the tortilla with the oil and sprinkle with the sea salt and herbs. Bake until crispy, approximately 10 minutes.

As the tortilla bakes, combine the avocado, lime juice, and mayonnaise. Remove the tortilla from the oven and spread the mixture on top before serving.

SESAME CHICKEN STIR-FRY

PHASE 3

Serves 4 to 6

1 to 1½ pounds organic skinless, boneless chicken breast
4 tablespoons toasted sesame oil
½ cup chopped red onion
2 tablespoons minced garlic
1 tablespoon grated ginger
¼ teaspoon crushed red pepper flakes
1 teaspoon minced cilantro or dried parsley
1½ cups chopped cauliflower
1½ cups chopped zucchini
1½ cups shredded green cabbage
Sea salt
Freshly ground black pepper
¼ cup toasted sesame seeds
2 to 3 cups cooked quinoa, warm

Cut the chicken into 1-inch pieces and set aside. Preheat a large nonstick skillet and add 3 tablespoons of the sesame oil. Sauté the onion for 5 to 7 minutes, until soft. Add the garlic and ginger, and sauté for another minute, until fragrant.

Add the chicken, the red pepper flakes, and cilantro to the skillet. Brown the chicken in the oil for a few minutes. Add broccoli and cook for 2 minutes. Add the zucchini and cabbage, and stir-fry until vegetables are the desired tenderness. If needed, add another tablespoon of sesame oil.

Add sea salt and pepper to taste. Sprinkle with toasted sesame seeds and serve over cooked quinoa.

COCONUT CURRY CHICKEN

PHASE 3
Serves 4

1 tablespoon olive oil
1 medium onion, diced
1 teaspoon sea salt
2 teaspoons curry powder
14-ounce can coconut milk*
1 cup canned diced tomatoes
2 tablespoons tomato paste
1 pound boneless, skinless organic chicken breast, cut into 1-inch cubes
3 packed cups baby spinach
2 cups cooked quinoa, warm

Heat the oil in a large skillet. Add the onion and salt, and sauté over medium heat for about 7 minutes, until translucent. Add the curry powder and sauté for an additional minute, until the spice fully coats the onion.

Incorporate the coconut milk, tomatoes, and tomato paste into the mixture. Stir occasionally for 5 minutes, until sauce slightly thickens. Fold in the chicken and simmer for 5 to 6 minutes, or until cooked through.

Stir the spinach into the mixture and cook for 3 minutes or until wilted.

Add a pinch more salt to taste, if needed.

Serve warm over the quinoa.

*In this recipe, coconut milk counts as your Phase 3 fruit.

CHICKEN AND QUINOA RISOTTO

PHASE 3
Serves 6

1½ pounds boneless, skinless chicken tenders
4 tablespoons olive oil
1 small onion, thinly sliced

1 red bell pepper, cored, seeded and thinly sliced
1 yellow bell pepper, cored, seeded, and thinly sliced
5 garlic cloves, thinly sliced
Sea salt
Freshly ground black pepper
4 tablespoons hummus
3 cups cooked quinoa
20 leaves fresh basil, cut in chiffonade

Cut the chicken into 1-inch pieces and set aside.

In a large nonstick skillet, heat the olive oil. Add the chicken and sauté for 5 minutes, or until golden brown.

Add the onion and bell peppers. Sauté for 1 or 2 more minutes. Add the garlic and sauté until the peppers become slightly limp but are still brightly colored, about 1 or 2 more minutes. Season to taste with salt and pepper. Remove the pan from the heat.

Stir in the hummus. Add the quinoa and basil, and toss until the basil is wilted. Serve hot.

SESAME CHICKEN AND RICE

PHASE 3

Serves 6

This rice dish is a great way to use up leftover cooked grains. You can use any phase-appropriate grain for this recipe.

1½ pounds boneless, skinless chicken thighs, chopped into 2-inch cubes
2 tablespoons toasted sesame oil
½ cup chopped red onion
1 tablespoon Simply Organic seasoning (mixture of sea salt, mustard, celery seed, garlic, onion, chile peppers, and black pepper) or a similar seasoning that you like
1 tablespoon minced garlic

3 cups trimmed and quartered Brussels sprouts
3 cups cherry tomatoes, halved
½ cup chopped fresh basil
3 teaspoons toasted sesame seeds

RICE
2 cups cooked wild rice
1 cup cooked black barley
1 tablespoon toasted sesame oil

Rinse the chicken and pat dry. Brown it in a large skillet with the sesame oil, onion, seasoning, and garlic. Continue to cook over medium heat until cooked through. Transfer the chicken to a holding plate. Set aside.

In the same pan, add the Brussels sprouts and stir-fry for approximately 1 to 2 minutes. Add the tomatoes and basil, and stir-fry for an additional 1 to 2 minutes.

Meanwhile, for the rice sauté all the grains in the oil. Keep warm.

Add the chicken to the skillet again and stir-fry everything for another 3 to 5 minutes, until the vegetables are cooked to the desired consistency. Sprinkle with the toasted sesame seeds and serve over ½ cup of rice medley.

BAKED SALMON AND SWEET POTATOES

PHASE 3

Serves 1

This recipe can be easily multiplied to serve as many as you like.

1 sweet potato
6 ounces wild-caught salmon fillet
Olive oil
¼ cup lemon juice
¹/₈ teaspoon sea salt

Crushed red pepper flakes to taste
½ teaspoon onion and/or garlic powder

Preheat the oven to 400 degrees. Wash the sweet potato and put on the oven rack. Bake for about 1 hour or until easily pierced with a fork. Keep oven set at 400 degrees.

Spray or lightly brush the salmon with olive oil. Sprinkle with the lemon juice and seasonings. Bake for 15 minutes, then transfer to broiler for 5 to 7 minutes. Serve with the potato.

AVOCADO CHILI

PHASE 3

Serves approximately 4

Because this recipe contains a large amount of starchy legumes, it counts as a Grain as well as a Protein and Veggie serving. No need to add an additional Grain, even if the meal map specifies a Grain.

1 pound lean ground turkey (or buffalo meat), browned and drained
½ cup chopped red onions
2 heaping tablespoons chili powder
2 tablespoons minced garlic
2 tablespoons parsley or cilantro
1 teaspoon crushed red pepper flakes (optional)
15-ounce can white beans or kidney beans
15-ounce can black beans or pinto beans
15-ounce can lentils or adzuki beans
4 medium zucchini, chopped
4 cups (32 ounces) red bell pepper tomato soup or tomato soup
1 heaping teaspoon sea salt
2 avocados, diced

Put meat, onions, chili powder, garlic, parsley or cilantro, and crushed red pepper flakes into a slow cooker on high.

Cover and set aside while prepping the remaining ingredients.

Open and drain all cans of beans. Add the beans, zucchini, and the soup to the pot and stir well.

Cook on high for 4 to 5 hours, or low for 6 to 8 hours.

Stir and taste occasionally, adjusting seasonings as needed.

Add the sea salt just before serving to preserve its nutrients.

Serve with diced avocado.

ROSEMARY PORK ROAST WITH SWEET POTATO

PHASE 3

Serves 8

2 pounds boneless pork loin
2 tablespoons olive oil
½ tablespoon sea salt
½ teaspoon black pepper
½ teaspoon dried rosemary
½ teaspoon dried thyme
¼ teaspoon dried sage
6 garlic cloves
8 small or 4 large sweet potatoes

Rub the pork with the olive oil, salt, pepper, rosemary, thyme, and sage. Using a knife, make slits in the roast and insert the garlic cloves.

Put the roast in a slow cooker. Halve the sweet potatoes and place them around and on top of the pork roast (not underneath, as they won't cook as well). Cook on low for 8 to 10 hours or on high for 6 to 8 hours.

SHRIMP AND VEGGIE STIR-FRY WITH QUINOA

PHASE 3

Serves 4

2 tablespoons olive oil

½ cup chopped red onion

3 teaspoons crushed garlic

12 to 14 asparagus stalks, trimmed and chopped

1½ to 2 cups quartered Brussels sprouts

3 teaspoons chopped cilantro

1 teaspoon crushed red pepper flakes

½ teaspoon sea salt

2 heads baby bok choy, bottoms removed

1 pound extra-large cooked shrimp

2 cups cooked quinoa, warm, or wild rice

Heat the olive oil in a large nonstick skillet. Stir-fry the onion for 4 minutes over medium heat. Add the garlic and sauté for another minute. Add the asparagus, sprouts, cilantro, red pepper flakes, and sea salt. Stir-fry until the vegetables are crisp-tender.

Add the bok choy and shrimp and continue to cook on medium-high heat until the shrimp is heated through.

Serve over quinoa or wild rice.

COCONUT PECAN-CRUSTED HALIBUT WITH ARTICHOKE AND DIP

PHASE 3

Serves 1

Olive oil spray

¼ cup crushed pecans

¼ cup shredded coconut

1 egg white

5 drops liquid Stevia

6 ounces halibut fillet
1 medium artichoke

DIP
1 teaspoon hummus
1 teaspoon lemon juice
1 teaspoon toasted sesame oil
Sea salt
Black pepper

Preheat the oven to 400 degrees. Cover a baking pan with aluminum foil and spray lightly with olive oil. Set aside.

In a small mixing bowl, combine the pecans and coconut. In another bowl, whip the egg white with a fork and add the Stevia. Dip the fish in the egg white, then roll it in the mixture, heavily coating the fish. Place the fish on the foil. Bake for approximately 20 minutes.

While fish is cooking, bring a pot of water to a boil. Wash the artichoke and remove the base. Cut in half lengthwise. When water is at a rolling boil, add the artichoke and boil until you can easily pull a leaf off with tongs, approximately 10 minutes. Drain. Prepare the dip by combining all ingredients in a small bowl.

Serve the fish with the artichoke, with dip alongside.

ALMOND BUTTER–STUFFED CELERY
PHASE 3
Serves 1

2 celery stalks
2 tablespoons almond butter
Coconut flakes or carob chips (optional)

Wash and clean the celery stalks. Cut into 2- to 3-inch pieces. Fill the celery pieces with the almond butter. Sprinkle with coconut flakes and/or carob chips.

THE FAST METABOLISM DIET

NUTTY JICAMA WITH LIME

PHASE 3

Serves 1

½ cup diced peeled jicama
¼ cup raw pine nuts
½ lime, juiced
Pinch of sea salt

Place the jicama in a small bowl. Add the pine nuts. Squeeze lime juice onto the jicama and pine nuts. Add salt and stir well.

WHITE BEAN AND DILL HUMMUS

PHASE 3

Serves 6

2 16-ounce cans chickpeas, drained, reserving ⅓ cup liquid
15-ounce can organic white beans
½ cup tahini
½ cup fresh lemon juice
1 to 1½ teaspoons sea salt
½ garlic clove
1 teaspoon dill
6 cups sliced cucumbers

Using a food processor or blender, blend the first seven ingredients together until smooth.

Serve each serving of hummus with 1 cup of sliced cucumbers.

CREAMY GUACAMOLE

PHASE 3

Serves 1

1 teaspoon safflower mayonnaise
½ avocado
1 teaspoon cilantro
1 teaspoon lime juice
⅛ teaspoon cracked red pepper
Salt and pepper to taste
1 cup sliced cucumber or jicama

Mash first 6 ingredients together and serve with sliced cucumber or ji-cama.

SWEET POTATO HUMMUS AND CUCUMBERS

PHASE 3

Serves 6

2 16-ounce cans chickpeas, drained, reserving ⅓ cup liquid
½ cooked sweet potato
½ cup tahini
½ cup fresh lemon juice
1 to 1½ teaspoons kosher salt
½ garlic clove
¼ teaspoon ground cumin
6 cups sliced cucumbers

Using a food processor or blender, blend all ingredients except cucumbers until smooth.

Serve each serving of hummus with 1 cup of sliced cucumbers.

CHAPTER TWELVE

HAYLIE
POMROY

The Super-Simple Diet Option

I always encourage you to cook, if possible, because I think cooking is fun and is a lot easier than most people think—and its health benefits are so worthwhile. If you really don't like to cook, or you truly don't have the time to cook but you want the convenience of grab-and-go foods, then this next option is for you.

The Super-Simple Diet Option uses my phase-specific Fast Metabolism Diet (FMD) breakfast shakes for *breakfast* each day (at ShopHayliePomroy .com). Each *morning snack* is the same during each phase, so these are easy to buy and stash. *Lunch* uses either leftovers from your dinner the night before or simple sandwiches and salads you can make in minutes. The phase-specific food bars (also available at ShopHayliePomroy.com) make every *afternoon snack* simple—just keep them in your desk or purse.

Finally, for *dinner*, this super-simple plan requires that you cook just seven slow cooker meals, which you can make the first week and then freeze for the rest of the weeks, taking you through the full 28 days.

SUPER-SIMPLE MEAL MAP, *PHASE 1*

PHASE 1: UNWIND STRESS

WAKE TIME	WEIGHT	BREAKFAST	SNACK	LUNCH	SNACK	DINNER	EXERCISE	WATER
__:__ am/pm **MONDAY**	———	__:__ am/pm P1 FMD BREAKFAST SHAKE	__:__ am/pm 1 APPLE	__:__ am/pm ½ TURKEY SANDWICH WITH SLICED NITRATE-FREE TURKEY, LETTUCE, CUCUMBER, TOMATO, AND MUSTARD	__:__ am/pm P1 FMD FOOD BAR	__:__ am/pm P1 CHILI		
__:__ am/pm **TUESDAY**	———	__:__ am/pm P1 FMD BREAKFAST SHAKE	__:__ am/pm 1 APPLE	__:__ am/pm CHILI AND 1 ORANGE	__:__ am/pm P1 FMD FOOD BAR	__:__ am/pm P1 CHICKEN AND BROCCOLI BOWL		

SUPER-SIMPLE MEAL MAP, *PHASE 2*

PHASE 2: UNLOCK FAT

WAKE TIME	WEIGHT	BREAKFAST	SNACK	LUNCH	SNACK	DINNER	EXERCISE	WATER
__:__ am/pm **WEDNESDAY**	_____	__:__ am/pm P2 FMD BREAKFAST SHAKE	__:__ am/pm NITRATE-FREE JERKY	__:__ am/pm SLICED TURKEY, MUSTARD, AND LETTUCE WRAP	__:__ am/pm P2 FMD FOOD BAR	__:__ am/pm P2 BEEF AND CABBAGE SOUP		
__:__ am/pm **THURSDAY**	_____	__:__ am/pm P2 FMD BREAKFAST SHAKE	__:__ am/pm NITRATE-FREE JERKY	__:__ am/pm LEFTOVER P2 BEEF AND CABBAGE SOUP	__:__ am/pm P2 FMD FOOD BAR	__:__ am/pm P2 PEPPERONCINI PORK ROAST		

SUPER-SIMPLE MEAL MAP, *PHASE 3*

						PHASE 3: UNLEASH YOUR METABOLISM		
WAKE TIME	WEIGHT	BREAKFAST	SNACK	LUNCH	SNACK	DINNER	EXERCISE	WATER
__:__ am/pm **FRIDAY**	____	__:__ am/pm P3 FMD BREAKFAST SHAKE	__:__ am/pm ¼ CUP RAW NUTS OR SEEDS	__:__ am/pm SALAD WITH TURKEY, TOMATO, CUCUMBER, AND AVOCADO, WITH P3 DRESSING	__:__ am/pm P3 FMD FOOD BAR	__:__ am/pm CURRY CHICKEN		
__:__ am/pm **SATURDAY**	____	__:__ am/pm P3 FMD BREAKFAST SHAKE	__:__ am/pm ¼ CUP RAW NUTS OR SEEDS	__:__ am/pm LEFTOVER P3 COCONUT CHICKEN CURRY	__:__ am/pm P3 FMD FOOD BAR	__:__ am/pm P3 SHRIMP VEGGIE STIR-FRY WITH RICE PASTA		
__:__ am/pm **SUNDAY**	____	__:__ am/pm P3 FMD BREAKFAST SHAKE	__:__ am/pm ¼ CUP RAW NUTS OR SEEDS	__:__ am/pm LEFTOVER P3 SHRIMP AND VEGGIE STIR-FRY OVER SALAD GREENS	__:__ am/pm P3 FMD FOOD BAR	__:__ am/pm P3 SESAME CHICKEN STIR-FRY		

Just use this meal map during the four weeks. Set aside one or two weekend days to make all the slow cooker meals. Then freeze them in individual portions for easy defrosting. Although I own three slow cookers myself, I've been known to borrow a friend's and get it all done in one night.

Sure, this plan contains less variety, but for many of my clients, the simplicity and convenience are well worth it.

Master Food Lists

This is a master list that includes every food you can eat for every phase. Whenever you need to know if it's okay to eat something within your phase, or if you are just looking for what to buy at the store for your phase, look here. Remember, whenever possible, choose organic.

PHASE 1 FOOD LIST
(select organic whenever possible)

VEGETABLES AND SALAD GREENS (FRESH, CANNED, OR FROZEN)

Arrowroot

Arugula

Bamboo shoots

Beans: green, yellow (wax), French

Beets

Broccoli florets

Cabbage, all types

Carrots

Celery, including tops

Cucumbers

Eggplant

Green chiles

Green onions

Jicama

Kale

Leeks

Lettuce (any except iceberg)

Lima beans

Mixed greens

Mushrooms

Onions, red and yellow

Parsnips

Peas: snap, snow

Peppers: bell, pepperoncini

Pumpkin

Rutabaga

Spinach

Spirulina

Sprouts

Sweet potatoes/ yams

Tomatoes

Turnips

Zucchini and winter or yellow summer squash

FRUITS (FRESH OR FROZEN)

Apples

Apricots

Asian pears

Berries: blackberries, blueberries, mulberries, raspberries

Cantaloupe

Cherries

Figs

Grapefruit

Guava

Honeydew melon

Kiwis

Kumquats

Lemons

Limes

Loganberries

Mangos

Oranges

Papaya

Peaches

Pears

Pineapples

Pomegranates

Strawberries

Tangerines

Watermelon

ANIMAL PROTEIN

Beef: filet, lean ground

Buffalo meat, ground

Chicken: skinless, boneless white meat

Corned beef

Deli meats, nitrate-free: turkey, chicken, roast beef

Game: partridge, pheasant

Guinea fowl

Haddock fillet

Halibut: fillet, steak

Pollock fillet

Pork: tenderloin

Sardines, packed in water

Sausages, nitrate-free: turkey, chicken

Sole fillet

Tuna, solid white, packed in water

Turkey: breast meat, lean ground

Turkey bacon: nitrate-free

VEGETABLE PROTEIN

Black-eyed peas

Chana dal/lentils

Chickpeas/garbanzo beans

Dried or canned beans: adzuki, black, butter, great northern, kidney, lima, navy, pinto, white

Fava beans, fresh or canned

BROTHS, HERBS, SPICES, AND CONDIMENTS

Brewer's yeast

Broths: beef, chicken, vegetable*

Dried herbs: all types

Fresh herbs: all types

Garlic, fresh

Ginger, fresh

Horseradish, prepared

Ketchup, no sugar added, no corn syrup

Mustard: prepared, dry

Natural seasonings: Bragg Liquid Aminos, coconut amino acids, tamari

Noncaffeinated herbal teas or Pero

Pickles, no sugar added

Salsa

Seasonings: black and

*Note: All broths, if possible, should be free of additives and preservatives.

white peppers, chili powder, cinnamon, crushed red pepper flakes, cumin, curry powder, nutmeg, onion salt, raw cacao powder, sea salt, Simply Organic seasoning

Sweeteners: Stevia, Xylitol (birch only)

Tomato paste

Vanilla or peppermint extract

Vinegar: any type

GRAINS AND STARCHES

Amaranth

Arrowroot

Barley

Brown rice: rice, cereal, crackers, flour, pasta, tortillas

Brown rice cheese or milk

Buckwheat

Kamut: bagels

Millet

Nut flours

Oats: steel-cut

Quinoa

Rice milk, plain

Spelt: pasta, pretzels, tortillas

Sprouted-grain: bagels, bread, tortillas

Tapioca

Teff

Triticale

Wild rice

HEALTHY FATS

None for this phase

PHASE 2 FOOD LIST
(select organic whenever possible)

VEGETABLES AND SALAD GREENS (FRESH, CANNED, OR FROZEN)

Arrowroot

Arugula

Asparagus

Beans: green, yellow (wax), French (string)

Broccoli florets

Cabbage, all types

Celery

Collard greens

Cucumbers, any type

Endive

Fennel

Green chiles, jalapeños

Green onions

Jicama

Kale

Leeks

Lettuce (any except iceberg)

Mixed greens

Mushrooms

Mustard greens

Onions, red and yellow

Peppers: bell, pepperoncini

Rhubarb

Shallots

Spinach

Spirulina

Swiss chard

Watercress

FRUITS (FRESH OR FROZEN)

Lemons

Limes

ANIMAL PROTEIN

Beef, all lean cuts: filet, tenderloin, strip, sirloin, shell steak, London broil, round steak, rump roast, stew meat, lean ground

Buffalo meat

Chicken: boneless, skinless white meat

Cod/scrod fillet

Corned beef

Deli meats, nitrate-free: roast beef, chicken, turkey

Dory fish fillet

Eggs, whites only

Flounder fillet

Game: venison, ostrich, elk

Halibut fillet

Jerky, nitrate-free: beef, buffalo, turkey, elk, ostrich

Lamb, lean cuts

Oysters, packed in water

Pork: loin roast, tenderloin

Salmon: nitrate-free smoked

Sardines, packed in water

Sole fillet

Tuna, packed in water

Turkey: breast steaks, lean ground

Turkey bacon: nitrate-free

VEGETABLE PROTEIN AND STARCHES
None this phase

BROTHS, HERBS, SPICES, AND CONDIMENTS

Brewer's yeast

Broths: beef, chicken, vegetable*

Dried herbs: all types

Fresh herbs: all types

Garlic, fresh, powdered

Ginger, fresh

Horseradish, prepared

Mustard: prepared, dry

Natural seasonings: Bragg Liquid Aminos, coconut amino acids, tamari

Noncaffeinated herbal teas or Pero

Pickles, no sugar added

Seasonings: black and white peppers, cayenne, chili powder, chili paste, chipotle, cinnamon, crushed red pepper flakes, cumin, curry powder, nutmeg raw cacao powder, onion salt, sea salt

Sweeteners: Stevia, Xylitol (birch only)

Tabasco

Vanilla or peppermint extract

Vinegar, any type (except rice)

GRAINS
None this phase

HEALTHY FATS
None this phase

*Note: All broths, if possible, should be free of additives and preservatives.

PHASE 3 FOOD LIST

(select organic whenever possible)

VEGETABLES AND SALAD GREENS (FRESH, CANNED, OR FROZEN)

Arrowroot

Artichokes

Arugula

Asparagus

Avocados

Bean sprouts

Beans: green, yellow (wax), French (string)

Beets: greens, roots

Bok choy

Broccoli

Brussels sprouts

Cabbage, all types

Carrots

Cauliflower florets

Celery

Chicory (curly endive)

Collard greens

Cucumbers

Eggplant

Endive

Fennel

Green chiles

Green onions

Hearts of palm

Jicama

Kale

Kohlrabi

Leeks

Lettuce (any except iceberg)

Mixed greens

Mushrooms

Okra

Olives, any type

Onions

Peppers: bell, pepperoncini

Radishes

Rhubarb

Seaweed

Spinach

Spirulina

Sprouts

Sweet potatoes/ yams

Tomatoes, fresh and canned: round, plum, cherry

Watercress

Zucchini and winter or yellow summer squash

FRUITS (FRESH OR FROZEN)

Blackberries

Blueberries

Cherries

Cranberries

Grapefruit

Lemons

Limes

Peaches

Plums

Prickly pears

Raspberries

ANIMAL PROTEIN

Beef: filet, steaks, lean ground

Buffalo meat

Calamari

Chicken: boneless, skinless dark or white meat, ground

Clams

Corned beef

Crab, lump meat

Deli meats, nitrate-free: turkey, chicken, roast beef

Eggs, whole

Game: pheasant

Halibut fillet

Herring

Lamb

Liver

Lobster meat

Oysters

Pork: chops, loin roast

Rabbit

Salmon, fresh, frozen, or nitrate-free smoked

Sardines, packed in olive oil

Sausage, nitrate-free: chicken, turkey

Scallops

Sea bass fillet

Shrimp

Skate

Trout

Tuna, packed in water or oil

Turkey

Turkey bacon: nitrate-free

VEGETABLE PROTEIN

Almond milk, unsweetened, almond cheese, almond flour

Cashew milk

Chickpeas/ garbanzo beans

Dried (or canned) beans: adzuki, black, butter, cannellini, Great Northern, kidney, lima, navy, pinto, white

Hemp milk, unsweetened

Lentils

GRAINS

Barley, black or white

Oats: steel-cut, old-fashioned

Quinoa

Sprouted-grain: bread, bagels, tortillas

Wild rice

BROTHS, HERBS, SPICES, CONDIMENTS, AND SUPPLEMENTS

Brewer's yeast

Broths: beef, chicken, vegetable*

Carob chips

Dried herbs: all types

Fresh herbs: all types

Garlic, fresh

Ginger, fresh

Horseradish, prepared

Ketchup, no sugar added, no corn syrup

Mustard, prepared, dry

Natural seasonings: Bragg Liquid Aminos, coconut amino acids, tamari

Noncaffeinated herbal teas or Pero

Pickles, no sugar added

Salsa

Seasonings: black and white peppers, cinnamon, chili powder, crushed red pepper flakes, cumin, curry powder, onion

salt, raw cacao powder, turmeric, sea salt, Simply Organic seasoning

Sweeteners: Stevia, Xylitol (birch only)

Tomato paste

Tomato sauce, no sugar added

Vanilla or peppermint extract

Vinegar, any type (except rice)

HEALTHY FATS

Avocados

Coconut, coconut milk, cream, water

Hummus

Mayonnaise, safflower

Nuts, raw: almonds, cashews, hazelnuts, pecans, pine nuts, pistachios, walnuts

Nut/seed butters and pastes, raw

Oils: coconut, grapeseed, olive, sesame, toasted sesame (Asian)

Seeds, raw: flax, hemp, pumpkin, sesame, sunflower

Tahini

*Note: All broths, if possible, should be free of additives and preservatives.

ACKNOWLEDGMENTS

I want to give special thanks to my agent, Alex Glass, who saw it all way before I could have even imagined it and to my invaluable attorney, John Fagerholm, who has always made sure I crossed my eyes and dotted my t's. I want to thank my friend and exceptionally talented producer Mason Novick, who told me I should write a book and then introduced me to the right people to make it happen.

A heartfelt thank-you to my incredibly understanding and creative editors, Talia Krohn and Heather Jackson (aka the closer), for being open to working outside the box because that is where I was comfortable.

I am so honored that two outstanding women, Tina Constable and Maya Mavjee, believed in my vision of creating a healthy way to lose weight while falling in love with food and bringing families and friends together around the dinner table again—forever I thank you. My entire team at Crown, especially Leigh Ann Ambrosi, Meredith McGinnis, and Tammy Blake, have been so patient and kind all the while driving the cause in just the right direction. I am in awe and so thankful for all you do.

I am so grateful to Eve Adamson, for it is amazing to work with a writer who gets you, your voice, and your twisted sense of humor. And to my coach Melanie, what a wild ride right? I cannot thank you enough.

Thank you to Larry Vincent and Michellene DeBonis at UTA for their amazing design and branding and most of all for really getting me.

And to my beloved Kim and Kym, I wouldn't be without either of you.

Thank you for jumping right in, being so generous, and egging me on all the way. To my dear friends Tim and Wendy, for feeding me and caring for me so I had the energy to feed and care for others, and to Chris and Karen for expanding my horizon beyond my wildest imagination and affirming that dyslexia is a reason to be successful and not that we find success despite it.

I want to thank all of my clients throughout the years. I have gained so much because you have allowed me into your lives and have shared with me your personal journeys. You know you hold a very special place in my heart.

I owe a special thanks to Colorado State University, specifically Dr. Nancy Irlbeck and Temple Grandin, for when I graduated I was so fired up to get out there and help people and make a difference in this world. And to Dr. Michael Towbin, Dr. Jackie Fields, and Dr. Orrie Clemens, thank you for mentoring me and integrating for the good of the patient.

To my sisters, Heather and Holli, you are my best friends and my rock in a storm or on a sunny day. Thank you for the late nights, for always being there for me, and for throwing me out there when I didn't think I could do it. Thank you for giving me Dolan and Harley for they are the real prize. To my dad, Nestor, I know I am your favorite and now it has been published as such and I love and thank you for being so good to me and the kids. My mom, Dr. Jeanne Wilson, you inspire every day to be a better mother, friend, and human being and I love you with all my heart.

I want to thank my amazing husband, Von, who swept in and unlocked all that was holding me back and keeping me down. With you I am home and you have blessed me with a rich and full family of five beautiful children. Thank you for reading and rereading and rereading chapter after chapter and telling me time and time again how smart and funny I was. Thank you for relocating all of Christmas in the middle of the night and remembering my passport and to turn out the horses and that I need my blanket when I fly and that sometimes sorbet and flowers do make everything better. And thank you for all the times you never asked me why. I love you. So many individuals and organizations are responsible for the actualization of this book and to you all I thank you from the bottom of my heart!

INDEX

Leek, Beef, and Kale Soup, 206
legumes, 78, 81, 105–7, 109. *See also* beans;
  lentils
lemonade, 87
lentils: Avocado Chili, 229–30
  Lentil Stew, 224
leptin, 20, 45
lettuce wraps. See sandwiches and wraps
lifestyle changes. See Fast Metabolism
  living
lipid panel, 44–45
liver health and function, 30, 34–35, 37,
  63, 87
  alcohol and, 94, 177, 179
  foods to support, 60, 63–64
  sugars and, 55
low-carb meals and diets, 66, 67–68,
  145
lunches, 121. *See also* meal maps
  Phase 1, 53, 59
  Phase 2, 61, 66–67
  Phase 3, 69, 75, 76
  timing, 86
lysine, 74

main courses: Phase 1, 184, 191–95
  Phase 2, 198–99, 208–12
  Phase 3, 216–17, 224–32
maintenance rules, 167–76
manahexolose, 73
mangos, 183
  Frozen Mango Fat-Burning Smoothie,
  184
massage, 69, 89, 128, 136, 138
meal maps, 116–17
  blanks, 118–21
  Super-Simple option, 235–39
  week one, 129–32
  week two, 138–42
  week three, 148–52
  week four, 155–61
meal timing, 18, 84, 85–86, 102–3
  after completing the diet, 169, 170
  Phase 1, 52–53, 56, 58–59
  Phase 2, 61, 66–67
  Phase 3, 69, 75–76
  skipping meals or snacks, 18–19, 85,
  136, 149, 178–79
measuring yourself, 109
meats, 88, 174. *See also* food lists; protein;
  specific types
  Phase 1, 56
  Phase 2, 62
menopause, 45

milk, 91. *See also* dairy foods
minerals, 37
mitochondria, 40, 54, 73, 173
muscle: fat burning and, 62, 63
  stress or starvation and, 18–19, 40
muscle development, 62, 63, 66, 92, 169
  acid levels and, 65
  exercise and, 148, 169
  Phase 3 toning, 74
mushrooms: Egg White, Mushroom, and
  Spinach Omelet, 200
  Stuffed Mushrooms, 215

nitrates, 88
norepinephrine, 92
nut butters, 88, 105–7
  Almond Butter-Stuffed Celery, 232
  B and B Toast, 217
nutrient density, 25
nutritional supplements, 174
nuts and seeds, 73, 74, 215. *See also*
  specific types
Berry Nutty Oatmeal, 219–20

oatmeal: Berry Nutty Oatmeal, 219–20
  Berry Nutty Oatmeal Smoothie, 219
  gluten-free, 111
  Oatmeal, 185
  Oatmeal Fruit Smoothie, 185
obesogens, 29
oils, 73, 105–7, 108, 245. *See also* fat,
  dietary; food lists
Olive and Tomato Salad, 222
olive oil, 73
omega-3 fatty acids, 74
omelets. See eggs
organic foods, 87, 174
organic wine, 177
oysters: Oysters Canapé, 214
  Oysters on the Half Shell, 214

pancreas, 55, 64, 70
parties. See special events
pasta: Chicken Sausage with Brown Rice
  Fusilli, 192–93
peanut butter, 88
pecans:
  Coconut Pecan-Crusted Halibut with
  Artichoke and Dip, 231–32
peppers: Chicken and Quinoa Risotto,
  226–27
  Pepperoncini Pork Roast, 212